Sand Therapy for Out of Control Sexual Behavior, Shame, and Trauma

This book is designed to educate sex therapists and mental health professionals on the power of using sand when treating sexual issues, providing guidance in accessing their clients' unconscious to seek new ways of healing.

Uniquely integrating sex therapy with sand therapy, Dawson describes how understanding and applying non-pathological theories and neuroscience to different modalities, such as Internal Family Systems and Polyvagal Theory, can help clients move forward from shame, sexual dysfunctions, and trauma. The book begins by introducing how therapists can use sand as a doorway into using metaphor and imagery in their practice, with information on how the nervous system keeps somatic experiences trapped in the body being explored. Written in an easy, accessible style, the book also includes case studies throughout to help therapists see the benefits of using sand with clients in practice.

Including forewords by Dr. Lorraine Freedle and Doug Braun-Harvey, this book is geared toward all mental health professionals, such as sex therapists and marriage and family therapists, who are working with individuals and couples seeking treatment for complex trauma and mental and sexual health issues. It will appeal to students as well as advanced mental health clinicians looking to expand their therapeutic tool kit.

Peg Hurley Dawson, Ph.D. is a psychotherapist who specializes in sexual health, problematic sexual behavior, sexual dissatisfactions, and complex trauma. She is a registered sandplay practitioner and creator of the IFSsandtray technique. She is affiliated with The American Association of American Sex Educators, Counsellors and Therapists, Society of Sex Therapy and Research, and Sandplay Therapists of America.

"If you are looking for a book that takes what we know about EMDR, IFS, Polyvagal Theory, and Sandplay and beautifully merges it with sex therapy and trauma, then this is definitely a book you must read. Dr. Peg Hurley Dawson takes the reader on a journey into the shadows of the subconscious mind using our "Parts" as the roadmap. This book is for any and all clinicians or anyone interested in the subconscious mind and healing. Have your highlighter and bookmarks ready because you'll be reading this over and over again."

Latina Edmonds, MA, LCMHC, CST, RYT

"In *Sand Therapy for Out of Control Sexual Behavior, Shame, and Trauma: Treatment Approaches Beyond Words*, Peg Dawson brilliantly integrates Internal Family Systems and Polyvagal Theory into her unique form of Sandtray Therapy. The product of her signature IFS Sandtray therapy is a powerful therapeutic strategy that provides a safe context for the 'parts' to have voice and to become integrated through an emergent healing process. By drawing from her extensive experience as a therapist, Dr. Peg Hurley Dawson builds vivid narratives providing examples of how challenged clients have been transformed through her insightful work to finally experience feelings of safety in another's arms."

Stephen W. Porges, PhD, Distinguished University Scientist,
Founding Director, Traumatic Stress Research Consortium,
Kinsey Institute, Indiana University Bloomington

Sand Therapy for Out of Control Sexual Behavior, Shame, and Trauma

Treatment Approaches Beyond Words

PEG HURLEY DAWSON

R Routledge
Taylor & Francis Group

NEW YORK AND LONDON

Designed cover image: © Getty Images

First published 2024
by Routledge
605 Third Avenue, New York, NY 10158

and by Routledge
4 Park Square, Milton Park, Abingdon, Oxon, OX14 4RN

Routledge is an imprint of the Taylor & Francis Group, an informa business

© 2024 Peg Hurley Dawson

Library of Congress Cataloging-in-Publication Data
Names: Hurley Dawson, Peg, author.
Title: Sand therapy for out of control sexual behavior, shame, and trauma :
treatment approaches beyond words / Peg Hurley Dawson.
Description: New York, NY : Routledge, 2024. | Includes bibliographical
references and index. |
Identifiers: LCCN 2023017855 (print) | LCCN 2023017856 (ebook) |
ISBN 9781032482903 (hardback) | ISBN 9781032482910 (paperback) |
ISBN 9781003388302 (ebook)
Subjects: MESH: Sexual Behavior--psychology | Play Therapy--methods |
Sexual Trauma--therapy | Sexual Dysfunctions, Psychological--therapy |
Psychotherapeutic Processes
Classification: LCC RC489.P7 (print) | LCC RC489.P7 (ebook) |
NLM WM 460.5.S3 | DDC 616.89/1653--dc23/eng/20230706
LC record available at https://lccn.loc.gov/2023017855
LC ebook record available at https://lccn.loc.gov/2023017856

ISBN: 9781032482903 (hbk)
ISBN: 9781032482910 (pbk)
ISBN: 9781003388302 (ebk)

DOI: 10.4324/9781003388302

Typeset in Dante and Avenir
by KnowledgeWorks Global Ltd.

For encouraging all people to embrace and accept who they are as unique individuals.
—Peg Hurley Dawson, PhD

Table of Contents

Acknowledgments

I am grateful to have an opportunity to give appreciation to individuals who supported me in this endeavor. I doubt this book would ever have materialized if our paths never crossed. It feels to me to have been a synchronistic journey. Each client started their expedition with me knowing my therapeutic style is very different from the therapists they had been to before. They trusted in an unknown process, of which some were very skeptical, but they desired healing over skepticism and gave it a try anyway.

It would be wonderful if I could name my clients without their pseudonyms, as each of them started their journey with me. I want to thank them first. Betty, Jane, Billy, John, and the others who wanted to share their experiences, are featured in Chapters 16 and 17.

Douglas Moser, editor, and coach has been with me and was a gift to my experience of the writer's voyage with all the challenges of any new adventure. Of course, I never would have met Doug if it wasn't for Dr. Tammy Nelson's writing and publishing class which ultimately changed my life.

My colleagues who walked the path with me, Dr. Yvonne Makidon, LaTina Edmonds, Chelsey Luke, Ethan Wattley, and Kim Denney inspired me with their comments and critiques of early manuscripts. In addition, I want to thank Theresa Valendzas, an IFS colleague, whose sense of humor I cherish.

My mentors Doug Braun-Harvey, Dr. Lorraine Freedle, and Sally Sugatt, all-wise beings place in my life and my gratitude for them is never ending. In addition, a few mentors I don't know personally, but they influenced me in my learning, Dr. Stephen Porges, Dr. Gabor Mate, Dr. Bruce Perry, Dr. Jeffery Rediger, and other great teachers in my lifetime.

And lastly, endless gratitude to my husband, Adrian, who has witnessed my metaphorical metamorphosis from chrysalis to spreading my wings and enjoying the freedom of flight.

Foreword by Dr. Lorraine Freedle

C. G. Jung describes the individuation journey as the process of becoming who we are meant to be. During certain times in our lives, the call to enter this process can no longer be ignored. At the risk of being lost to ourselves forever, we must follow our soul's yearning to live authentically.

Jungian/Kalffian Sandplay Therapy (sandplay) is a primarily nonverbal and non-directive method of psychotherapy that can directly connect us to our deepest desires. Founded by Dora Kalff, Swiss psychotherapist and student of Carl Jung, sandplay has roots in Jungian theory, contemplative practices, and play therapy. In sandplay we use symbols, sand, our hands, and imagination to create our inner world in a tray of sand as an attuned therapist provides emotional safety and bears witness to our unfolding story. Much like an active dream, sandplay taps into conscious and unconscious dimensions of the psyche to help us access lost or hidden resources for healing and transformation. Sandplay provides the conditions necessary to naturally bring forth Jung's individuation journey.[1]

When I met the author of this book, Dr. Peg Hurley Dawson, she was already well-established in her career as a psychotherapist specializing in working with people who experienced complex developmental trauma as well as those with problem sexual behavior. She possessed great compassion for people of diverse backgrounds in need of emotional healing, including those who were disenfranchised and often marginalized by the dominant culture. She was grounded in the neurobiology of trauma and well-trained in several contemporary therapeutic approaches such as EMDR, Internal Family Systems (IFS), and Sensorimotor Psychotherapy. She also developed a unique way of expanding IFS with sandtray therapy.

Even with this remarkable level of training and expertise, Peg yearned to integrate sandplay into her practice. She searched for a mentor to help guide her through the training process. Robby Aikin, a mutual friend and esteemed colleague who shared our dedication to helping trauma survivors, encouraged Peg to contact me. To this day, I remain grateful to Robby for his trust and intuition in connecting us.

As soon as I met Peg, it became clear that she was extremely dedicated to her clients and was looking for more than a new method for her toolbox. Peg was answering her soul's calling for greater depth and wholeness—personally and professionally. She wanted to learn more about the unconscious and its role in the healing process. She wanted to revisit her past in a new way to overcome limiting beliefs. She was being called to travel further on her path toward authentic living so that she could carry forward the fruits of her labor to those she cares for in psychotherapy.

Peg rolled up her sleeves and did the work—in the sand, in the classroom, and in her professional life. This book is a product of years of training, development, and integration. Offering wisdom that is shared enthusiastically and generously, in the pages that follow Peg provides therapists with accessible knowledge, understanding, and strategies for creative psychotherapy practice across theories and applications including Polyvagal Theory, Internal Family Systems, and sand therapies.

… and beyond the words and concepts in this book, lie the courageous and layered journeys of healing and transformation. May these stories inspire all of us to chart our unique pathway toward becoming who we are meant to be.

Lorraine Razzi Freedle, Ph.D.
International Sandplay Teacher (STA/ISST)[2].

Notes

1 *Sandplay: A Psychotherapeutic Approach to the Psyche*, trans. Boris L. Matthews (Oberlin, OH: Analytical Psychology, 2020). (Original work published in 1966.)

2 Sandplay Therapists of America and the International Society for Sandplay Therapy.

Foreword by Doug Braun-Harvey

Peg Dawson invites fellow clinicians into her psychological toolkit of hope for healing complex trauma, mental health, and sexual health issues. This deeply client-centered integration offers a wide range of therapy modality tools for guiding clients in healing themselves. Dawson carefully builds a relationship with the reader as she constructs her assertion that it is indeed the client, unbeknownst to themselves, who brings their answers to our clinical rooms.

Reflecting on the book's detailed mapping of the connections between the physical and mental aspects of the Self, and methods for how a therapist engages with the many personality components of thoughts and emotions within us all (that you will learn to call "Parts"), I suddenly recalled a conference I attended in 2007.

The world's Spanish-speaking countries convened over four days in Bogotá, Columbia for the Pan-American Association Conference on the Prevention of Child Maltreatment. The participants included police officers, lawyers, judges, child abuse investigators, medical evaluators, therapists, social workers, and national leaders in child abuse prevention. My husband, Al Killen-Harvey, an internationally respected advocate and trainer for child abuse treatment professionals, and I, a trainer in group process and sexual health, gave a one-hour presentation on the final day of the conference. Our message, reflected by similar themes in this book, was that every interaction between an abused, neglected or violently harmed child and a child abuse services professional is an opportunity for therapeutic healing.

We had never before given a presentation that would be simultaneously translated over headphones worn by each attendee. In the days before our presentation, we noticed the English-speaking presenters talking at a rate of speech that did not take into consideration the delay resulting from translating their words into Spanish. The presenters moved on to their next slide while the headphone-equipped audience was laughing, sighing, or emotionally responding to the previous slide. We thought this was a missed opportunity for rapport with the audience. Failing to improvise and adjust to the Spanish language translation milieu led to a less attuned affinity with the audience, which was inconsistent with the conference goal of building professionals better attuned to serving maltreated children and their families.

Al and I spent the next two days strategizing and adjusting our presentation to reflect the simultaneous translation setting. We cut our content in half. We practiced speaking much, much more slowly (think of it like changing an iPhone podcast replay from 2X to 0.75X). We took our time between each question and comment to allow for translation.

We started by asking participants to raise their hands to identify as officers of the court, law enforcement personnel, medical providers, social workers, and therapists. About ten percent of the audience raised their hands when we asked: "How many of you are therapists?"

We spent the hour telling stories about how a police officer or an emergency room nurse or a receptionist at a clinic could be "a therapist" who provides a meaningful and soothing moment of attunement, a moment that a child will remember. It might be their warm facial expression, gentle comment, a kind gesture, or simply listening. We asserted that any one of these small moments has the potential to be a vital part of "therapy" in a child's healing journey. We invited them to consider the possibility of their conscious decision to attune with a child being stored in the child's body to be recalled at some later time. As Dawson explains so well, the many thinking Parts and emotional Parts contained within our personality store and manage early life memories as physical sensations, unconscious symbols and objects, all of which can be called upon later as keys for healing.

Al and I stood side by side on the stage taking turns to speak. When it was my turn, I slowly walked forward as Al took a few steps behind. This gentle choreographed flow between us settled our bodies. Our rate of speech remained slow and deliberate. As the hour progressed, we noticed many attendees removing their headsets. We were speaking English slowly enough for some to understand us without translation. We laughed together, we sighed together, we sat in quiet contemplation together.

In the closing minutes we paused, and slowly asked once again the same question: "How many of you are therapists?" Without delay, a thousand people silently, solemnly and in unison raised their hands. As I write this passage my body can still feel the electricity of that moment. As I remember the thousand hands proudly raised, my eyes water and feel a shiver of awe course through my body.

I searched through *Sand Therapy for Out of Control Sexual Behavior, Shame, and Trauma: Treatment Approaches Beyond Words* looking for clues that may have activated this memory of carefully calibrating all aspects of our presentation to the audience—a presentation itself focused on the crucial role of considered communication in healing. I was grateful to find in Chapter 7 the importance of a caretaker's responses to a child's actions and how the ways in which a caregiver responds forms a child's identity and core beliefs.

Peg Dawson's insightful work provides an invaluable framework for unpacking such moments. Her infectious enthusiasm, clarity, and confidence, as demonstrated in this remarkable book, deepen my understanding of what happened in our shared embodied states in Bogotá, as well as bringing informed biological and neurological explanations for my somatic sensations recalling this unforgettable training moment.

I am grateful to Peg Dawson for bringing us her scientific, practical and relational "experiential milieu" for clinicians to help their clients to find within themselves a restoration process that improves physical, mental, and sexual health. I am honored to see my original work in sexual health approaches for men with out of control sexual behavior adapted within this elegant integrative therapy method. *Sand Therapy for Out of Control Sexual Behavior, Shame, and Trauma: Treatment Approaches Beyond Words* artfully brings together Sandtray, Sandplay, Polyvagal Theory, Internal Family Systems (IFS) and Integrative Neuro Linguistic Programming (INLP), Default Mode Network (DMN), Neurosequential Model of Therapeutics (NMT) and innovative Pro-Symptom Belief Cards in an elegant therapist map for guiding clients to "delve deeper into the world of their personal as well as the collective unconscious, trusting in a process where the 'great unknown', the human psyche, is allowed to guide the journey to inner healing."

Each chapter encourages therapists to see beyond our limiting thoughts and emotions to find an opening to learn and change. You will be invited to move beyond talk therapy dialogues and join your clients in the sand as they introduce you to their personality of emotional and thought Parts, opening up new possibilities for their transformation and healing.

There are many fine gems to be found in this book, including exceptionally presented studies, neuroscience, clinical case examples and beautiful transcripts of a therapist documenting their in-session caretaking responses. Peg Dawson presents a wide range of clinical methods designed to suspend judgements and to discourage pathological labels and ill-timed evaluative opinions. I hope you find your curious mind stimulated and inspired by these innovative strategies that move beyond words, exploring the spaces that nurture the unconscious inner life of our clients, and perhaps our own as well.

Douglas Braun-Harvey, LMFT, CST, CST-S

Preface

Many people come to me to understand fully the whys behind their behavior. They're hoping to heal from complex trauma and other mental and sexual health issues. Some of their behaviors and emotional stressors include a lack of connection with their partner(s), sexual issues—including out of control or problematic sexual behavior, and attention deficit disorder (ADD). Several of these individuals have said to me, "I don't know if what you do is going to be able to help me. I have tried everything else with many other therapists." Or "My partner can't take my behavior anymore; I am out of control. They are going to leave me, and you're my last hope." Or even, "I have given up and don't think I can ever have sex again."

Some of these individuals experience physical restrictions causing them to experience sexual challenges such as pain with sex or erectile issues. The most important aspect of my work is helping them discover themselves in a new way. Often, I find the person's issues stem from childhood, how they were loved, treated, and how they learned to survive in their families of origin. Yes, survive. Human beings all have developed ways of coping in life, and it begins where we all started, with our families.

All human beings learn in their family of origin to take on certain roles that codify behavior. They become the jokester, or the fun one, the strong one, or the quiet one. Yet others are forced early in life to take on a parental role, which can lead them to a life of caretaking for others while neglecting their own needs. It may be hard to believe some even still suffer from the after effects of a major childhood illness, myself included. In Gabor Mate's 2003 book, *When the Body Says No: Exploring the Stress-Disease Connection,* he discusses how negative early childhood experiences can result in physical illnesses. He wrote,

> The biology of potential illnesses arise early in life. The brain's stress-response mechanisms are programmed by experiences beginning in infancy, and so are the implicit, unconscious memories that govern our attitudes and beviours toward ourselves, others, and the world. Cancer, multiple sclerosis, rheumatoid arthritis, and other conditions we examined are not abrupt new developments in adult life, but culminations of lifelong processes. The human interactions and biological imprinting that shaped these processes took place in periods of our life for which we may have no conscious recall.

As Mate stated above, my body said no when I was only seven. I became ill with a kidney disease where the doctors said to my parents I would either physically grow out of it or possibly it could end my life in my early teens. This made them pay a lot of attention to me, which I believe saved my life; unfortunately, I still was raised in chaos. By the age of twenty my body said no again, only this time it was thought of as a mental breakdown. I floundered for years in and out of therapy, some good others not so much. This was my introduction to the mental health care system. At that time—like most of the clients I see—when asked about my childhood history, I would reply "I had a great childhood." I was very lucky growing up on a farm with twenty-one acres of land, had all kind of animals that I loved, and had friends. Reflecting back, I can see how skewed my memory was, neglecting to mention my alcoholic father with anger issues. How could I have enjoyed a good and mentally healthy childhood?

I now know my experiences were the first steps along my path to becoming the therapist I am today. Some call those in the mental health field "wounded healers;" I believe this is often true. I have colleagues who have suffered from mis-attunement from their parents; or perhaps they grew up with a caretaker who was an alcoholic, depressed, or suffered from anxiety of some sort. I know countless health professionals who grew up in dysfunctional families like my own, resulting in them experiencing depression, anxiety, and other mental health issues where they sought therapy for themselves. The path to their healing also led them to help others heal.

Many times, it is in the therapeutic relationship, carefully forged by therapist and client, where healing happens. Relief is often found by working with an attuned and attentive non-judgmental professional trained in the art of psychological repair. There's no wonder many who have experienced successful treatment choose to study psychology themselves. I am an example of this. I had a degree in art and design and never thought in a million years I would become a therapist. But with years of being a client, I became so intrigued with the workings of the human mind that I wanted to explore it further. I went back to school to continue my studies, fully engaged in a pursuit of something deeper.

I recall a paper I wrote while studying for my master's in art therapy, in a class that introduced me Jungian Art Therapy. Carl Jung (1875–1961), himself a wounded healer, was mentored by Sigmund Freud. Both Freud and Jung shared an interest in the unconscious, although each viewed it differently, resulting in one of the reasons Freud terminated their relationship. Jung suffered great emotional distress over his separation and isolation from Freud and his adherents whereas Freud focused primarily on suppressed emotions and their impact on human behavior, Jung believed in the concept of the collective unconscious. The collective unconscious trusts that all human beings are connected to each other through shared experiences. While researching this paper, I learned just how much Jung's depression led him to the creative streak that would fuel his later work. I felt it parallel to my own experience of dealing with depression, anxiety, and my own belief of not being good enough.

This is where I first learned about the collective unconscious, and universal symbols, such as trees, sun, moon, and fire. Through metaphor, humans can express difficult situations or feelings. One example could be the metaphor "she/he has a heart of stone" which implies someone is mean, uncaring, or even cruel.

This leads to an understanding of how myths, fairytales, symbology, worldwide traditions, and analogies can be significant in art therapy. I learned about Jungian terms such as animus/anima, heaven/underworld, and many other concepts. All of this I use in my therapeutic practice to this day. Once I received my master's in art therapy, I began my own process with an art therapist and supervision with another art therapist supervisor. The drive to continue, to dig deeper into newer practices, continued. Art therapy opened up a new understanding for me, pointing me in the direction of learning more about other modalities.

Although I was indeed excelling in my craft as a new art therapist, I carried the belief that I wasn't good enough. I didn't realize, at that time, this very belief would ultimately become the driving force that would advance my career and my life. This belief made me want to take other advanced training in various modalities and techniques, all used in treating trauma. With each training, I hired a therapist who was well versed in that modality.

I would hire a supervisor to *really learn it*, and I would work towards certification so *I could master it*. I got certified in many of those modalities, one by one.

My first such undertaking was Eye Movement Desensitization and Reprocessing (EMDR) followed by Internal Family Systems (IFS), Ericksonian hypnosis, and other methods including Sensorimotor Psychotherapy. In addition, I became fascinated with human sexuality, so while learning the above modalities, I applied and received my certification in sex therapy from the American Association of Sex Educators, Counselors and Therapists (AASECT). As an AASECT sex therapist, when the time was right, I spent additional time training to become a supervisor by AASECT, a position I hold today.

I continued my education by training in the non-pathological lens of the Polyvagal Theory developed by Dr. Stephen Porges. The Polyvagal Theory (PVT) explains how the autonomic nervous system affects so many aspects lying underneath much of human behavior. This theory was helpful with my thinking around sexual issues, including out of control sexual or problematic sexual behavior, and other sexual issues, including the inability to experience sexual pleasure. This understanding of human responses, those that occur beneath the surface, led me to a whole new realm in my sex therapy and practice.

Many of my clients find me for treatment of "sex addiction," the quotation marks placed on the two words *sex* and *addiction* are intentional because of new insights in the treatment of OCSB or problematic sexual behavior. Doug Braun Harvey, LMFT, CGP, CST and Michael Vigorito, LMFT, LCPC, LCGP, authors of the 2016 book, *Treating Out of Control Sexual Behavior: Rethinking Sex Addiction*. This book introduces a non-judgmental based approach to treating OCSB. It is founded on the six sexual health principles which are based on the ethical rights by the World Health Organization. These principles are for consensual sexual behavior which takes into account consent, non-exploitation, honesty, shared values, mutual pleasure, and protection from HIV-STI's, and unwanted pregnancy.

For anyone who is involved in non-consensual sexual behavior, such as voyeurism, exhibitionism, or other non-consenting behaviors, a referral will be provided to another professional who specializes in non-consensual sexual behavior such as the Association for the Treatment of Sexual Abusers. www.atsa.com.

The field of sex therapy has been embroiled in a long-running debate between the sex therapists trained by the American Association of Sex Educators, Counselors, and Therapists, and the certified sex addiction therapists (CSAT) when referring to problematic or out of control sexual behavior.

The controversy lies mainly in the fact that CSATs label problematic sexual behavior as an addiction. This label has been proved detrimental and is often used in pathologizing people mistakenly diagnosed with mental health and sexual disorder diagnoses. Reframing it as problematic sexual behavior aligns it with a non-pathologizing lens, which is trauma informed. This information includes understanding how the autonomic nervous system influences emotions resulting in behaviors and how the brain developed from the brainstem up to the cortex is also critical.

I believe out of control or problematic sexual behavior is not a cycle of addiction, but of the fight or flight instinct, or sympathetic arousal of the autonomic nervous system (ANS). After studying the Polyvagal Theory, I realized how the ANS responds within milliseconds unconsciously causing the body to instantly prepare to react. In that exact moment mobilizing to deal with perceived or actual threats. There isn't any intentional or conscious thought in that millisecond, the body mobilized, and seeks regulation.

Through the work of Dr. Bruce Perry, I learned about the Neurosequential Model of Therapeutics (NMT) which is critical and important in understanding how our brains develop in childhood and later affects behaviors, such as sexuality in adulthood.

Healing childhood trauma can take decades to heal with traditional talk therapy. Early childhood trauma is directly related to the negative beliefs the word held persist well into adulthood. Often, I hear clients echo the very thoughts that plagued me: "I am not good enough," "I am damaged," as well as other negative core judgements. These beliefs cause many to suffer with insecurities. Causing individuals to compare themselves to others. They never dreamt it is possible to be in powerful positions. Even CEOs of Billion-dollar companies seek consultation or therapy as a result of situations which occurred in childhood, resulting in moments of insecurity years later. This book is different from books that rely on standard talk-based therapy, because it is about healing *without using words* and trusting in a process led by the unconscious.

There is one therapeutic modality that I've had tremendous success in accessing the unconscious, often without the use of words: Sandplay. Sandplay therapy has been around since the late 1950s, yet in 2023 most people haven't even heard of it. This book is intended to draw attention to this overlooked therapy. I have learned through both personal experience and in-depth study just how useful it is. It has, in short, shown me how I can trust in its process. Sandplay taught me to trust thinking in metaphor and the unconscious with all my clients. Through years of putting this into my practice, I have found this significant in assisting clients in their healing journeys.

Dr. Martin Kalff's description of the unconscious, elegantly composed in his 2022 book: *Old and New Horizons of Sandplay Therapy: Mindfulness and Neural Integration* he wrote,

> The personal unconscious comprises forgotten, repressed and dissociated contents, which used to be conscious at some point in life. Jung's view of the *personal* unconscious corresponds to the Freudian definition of the unconscious, meaning that it is of a personal nature and contains what Jung referred to as a 'feeling-toned complexes.' By contrast, the collective unconscious is not a personal acquisition and has never been conscious. Its contents are archaic imprints coming from a common human heritage, which Jung named 'archetypes.' Archetypes themselves represent the mind's tendency, similarly to instincts, and they do not have a specific form.

Although there are few registered sandplay practitioners (RSP) or certified sandplay therapists (CST) in the United States of America, sandplay is practiced all over the world. At the time this book was written in my state, Massachusetts, there were only three therapists listed who are trained in Kalffian Sandplay, a clinician in New Bedford, and another who practices in the western part of the state, and me. All of us are RSPs; the closest CST-T is in southern New Hampshire. The 'T' in CST-T denotes a teacher of Kalffian sandplay therapy.

I hope to inspire more therapists to incorporate sandplay or thinking in metaphor into their practice and their therapeutic tool kits. I hope to show how working with metaphor or sand to access the unconscious can become an integral component of the therapy. Many of my clients who healed with sandplay said it seemed to align with what they learn to identify as their Ego, with their souls. This is how Chapter 16 received the title, "Soul Reflections: Discovery of Self-Acceptance." This book was written with passion and is shared with you, the professional, who is also deeply vested and passionate about your work healing clients.

Comprehending how we all can accomplish this is covered within these pages. I have seen in my own personal experiences with the mental health system, and my own therapy, how a "diagnosis" can create its own stigma. Like many, what followed was a series of doctors and therapists, all working from the same prescriptive "rule book," citing references from the DSM. Despite the adherence to the rulebook, the therapies, and diagnosis contained in the DSM result in negative biases and pathological thinking by the professionals. Decades later, with thousands of dollars spent, I sought to understand this in new ways, partaking in cutting-edge modalities.

Over the years many clients told me they have been in therapy with a variety of different therapists. Each clinician was trained in specific modalities, and from those frameworks they worked on healing people using the methods they had in their therapeutic tool kits. They all took an oath when they received their licenses to practice therapy, to do no harm. And yet, many clients were, if not harmed, certainly not helped by the more traditional techniques. For them, therapy itself added to the trauma, rather than deliver them from their suffering. Certainly, there was room for something new, something innovative.

I have come to understand and know what is required to restore physical, mental, and sexual health lies within each of us. I have seen results again and again in my therapeutic practice with clients who work in the sand—or metaphor—and find healing. So much so, one of my clients recently said to me, "I was angry last week when we spent the entire session just talking and I didn't get to work in the sand." He had forgotten he asked me a complex question, wanted to know the answers, and needed clarification on certain details. It took more time than either of us expected it to and we didn't have enough time left to work in the sand.

I wrote this book to give hope where all hope is lost. I know this book will assist other healthcare professionals help their clients because it is not the therapist who is going to heal them. The therapist is only providing the tools so the clients can heal themselves. The answer is always in the room and it's never the clinician who comes up with it. The clients hold all the answers inside themselves; it is our job to help them discover it.

References

Braun-Harvey, D., & Vigorito, M., *Treating out of control sexual behavior: rethinking sex addiction.* Springer Publishing Company, LLC, New York, NY, 2016.

Kalff, M., *Old and new horizons of sandplay therapy: Mindfulness and neural integration.* Routledge, New York, NY, 2022.

Mate, G., *When the body says no: Exploring the stress-disease connection.* Turner Publishing, 2003.

How to Use This Book

Whether you are a student or have been in your professional role for thirty or more years, I suggest approaching this textbook with a beginner's mind. In many teachings, particularly from Eastern philosophy, the concept of a beginner's mind refers to a state of eagerness and openness when approaching new material. On the one hand, one holds the wisdom and knowledge that one has obtained over many years of existence but combines this with the ability to approach all new situations with the curiosity of a beginner. This allows one to learn new things and new ways of thinking that can be layered over existing knowledge and wisdom.

Many mental health professionals love their chosen careers, where they are instrumental in supporting individuals in shifting from feelings of despair, hopelessness, and loneliness to improved self-esteem, allowing them to live more full, productive lives. These professionals see profound transformations, in which their clients can embrace themselves—maybe for the first time—without shame, guilt, fear, and seeing them forward with confidence, clarity, and success.

This book is designed for both passionate clinicians entering the field and seasoned specialists, authorities, and experts who want to learn something new that will intrigue and challenge them. New information must be inspiring, interesting, and stimulating enough to motivate and enliven the most iconic leaders and thinkers in the field of psychotherapy. This textbook is brimming with thoughts from trailblazers who developed innovative and groundbreaking modalities to treat trauma, attachment wounds, and other mental or sexual health issues. The following pages and chapters you are about to read, are in themselves, unique and will integrate new concepts. While most textbooks focus only on one modality in the treatment of trauma, this textbook differs in that it integrates numerous empirically supported interventions from various clinically researched modalities.

Section One: Mapping Out the Journey.

I suggest you read these first eight chapters sequentially. The material detailed here provides a scaffolding for this textbook. Each segment contains a framework within itself, building a foundation of narratives which, when combined, become the groundwork and substance for the remaining chapters.

Chapter 1, **Introduction: Amazing Things Happen When You Trust the Process** focuses on exploring mental or sexual health issues with the latest up-to-date non-pathologizing treatments. These therapeutic methods work with the unconscious to heal those who suffer from problematic sexual behavior, both sexual and non-sexual shame, guilt, and trauma. Trauma symptomology frequently appears as anxiety, depression, or another diagnosis. Many mental health professionals continue to treat symptoms and don't address the underlying trauma. This chapter provides clarity in integrating neuroscience with creative therapeutic modalities, including play, which is rarely considered in the adult population.

Chapter 2, **Cutting-Edge Psychotherapy: Using Sand and Metaphor in Treatment** brings the concept of adding play into therapy with adults. Play stimulates the creative right hemisphere of the brain which brings the unconscious to consciousness solving issues the left hemisphere can't. Most talk therapies fail in comparison to this innovative approach. By working with sand and figurines, we could discover transformation, accessing the unconscious, resulting in the shift health care professionals have been seeking.

Chapter 3, **What Path to Choose? The Difference: Sandtray or Sandplay** informs both professionals unfamiliar with these two diverse modalities as well as those who currently use a sand tray with miniatures or figurines. Language matters, especially the terms of Sandtray or Sandplay therapy. Those who are trained in Sandplay know this immediately, but many others use the terms as if they are interchangeable. This is a mistake. This segment of the book clarifies the methods and techniques in these major influencing therapeutic modalities.

Chapter 4, **Innate Abilities to Navigate Difficult Terrain: Introduction to the Polyvagal Theory** was inspired by a session which took place with a client who experienced problematic sexual behavior. John, like so many others, suffered from a dysregulated autonomic nervous system (ANS), resulting in an explanation of how this aspect of his body developed its own built-in defense system. The ANS operates beneath the level of conscious awareness in the subcortical brain. Written in an easy-to-understand narrative, this chapter details how John, over the course of this session, walked away with hope. By understanding the role childhood trauma and the ANS played in his behavior.

Chapter 5, **Multiplicity: Introduction to Parts in Therapy** discusses two innovative psychotherapeutic constructs: Internal Family Systems (IFS) and Integrative Neuro Linguistic Programming (INLP), Both of these are patient-driven modalities that operate on the concept that the personality comprises of many thoughts and emotions called, "Parts." Again, an anecdote is used to explain and simplify the concepts. Integration of the Polyvagal Theory is applied in this chapter for even more clarity.

Chapter 6, **Adaptive Defenses to Use on the Journey: Using Internal Family Systems Through the Polyvagal Theory Lens** uses Joseph Campbell's concept of the hero's journey to observe how the non-pathological model of Internal Family Systems (IFS) and the Polyvagal Theory (PVT) protect psyche and body instantaneously, unconsciously, and within milliseconds. The chapter includes graphics and descriptions of emotions, identified as Parts in the IFS model with the physiological states of the autonomic nervous system in the PVT. The chapter explains how the ventral vagal state in PVT is like Self in IFS, Sympathetic arousal in PVT has characteristics of protective Parts known as Managers and Firefighters in IFS, and dorsal vagal can be considered Exiles in IFS.

Chapter 7, **What Goes in the Backpack? Impact of Early Childhood Trauma on Adult Sexuality** introduces the impact of early childhood trauma, which is often displayed in problematic sexual behavior and other sexual issues, shame, guilt, and core negative beliefs. Information on the Default Mode Network (DMN), how the brain forms from the brainstem up to the cortex, and the Neurosequential Model of Therapeutics (NMT) underscores the depth of childhood trauma. The NMT explores the impact of trauma on the young developing brain which ultimately affects people in adulthood. The NMT assists clinicians in the treatment of mental and sexual health issues, knowing which therapeutic modality to utilize, and design a comprehensive treatment plan.

Chapter 8, **Accessing the Unconscious Mind: Using Metaphor, Sandplay, and IFSsandtray** acquaints the reader with somatically held sensations, how the unconscious works in metaphor, and approaching therapeutic work with sand

and miniatures. This chapter informs the reader with research on integration of the Parts, Neurosequential Model of Therapeutics, and sandplay. It includes graphs and charts making it easy to review how the brain can heal when given a safe space and attuned therapist. This chapter also provides insight into how "playing" in the sand can help regulate the autonomic nervous system.

Section Two: "Courageous Souls Who Heal with In-Depth Therapy" uses real-life clients to illustrate the concepts discussed. Each chapter is either a case study or thorough description of one session with the following clients: Betty, Billy, and Jane.

Chapter 9, **Betty: Healing Early Childhood Trauma with the Pro-Symptom Belief Cards** explores one session with Betty who held the core negative belief she was inadequate. The session details how, by identifying her core negative belief, she could tap into various body sensations to heal three "wounded Parts," that held her back.

Chapter 10, **Billy: Problematic Sexual Behavior: Head Down, Holding Shameful Secrets** describes how Billy struggled in his marriage with a devastating secret that could potentially end his marriage if he ever told his wife. The chapter illustrates how, through a series of sessions, Billy could confront the motives behind his out of control sexual behavior.

Chapter 11, **Billy: Healing from Grief, Loneliness, and Out of Control Sexual Behavior with Sandplay** illustrates how Billy healed with the modality of Kalffian Sandplay. Photographs of fourteen out of thirty sandplay sessions are shown and discussed.

Chapter 12, **Jane: Letting Go of Painful Sex Through IFSsandtray** demonstrates a single IFSsandtray session where Jane meets the protective Part of herself that prevented her from experiencing penetrative sex. This session Jane learns how to communicate directly with her protective Part, listen to its messages and warnings, and within two weeks had intercourse with her partner four times without experiencing any pain.

Chapter 13, **Jane: Polarization of Shame and Being Sexually Free** reveals Jane's polarity of having two Parts, one that shamed her and the other that wanted to be sexually uninhibited. By integrating IFSsandtray into her therapy, Jane could understand how these Parts were working on two competing agendas.

Section Three: "Clinical Exercises"

Clinical Exercises, consists of two chapters, which also use real-life clients to illustrate how to do clinical exercises. Chapter 14 illustrated four sessions of utilizing Internal Family Systems Sandtray with Betty. Chapter 15 is two sessions utilizing the Pro-Symptom Belief Cards.

Chapter 14, **Internal Family Systems Directives to Use with Clients** describes two Internal Family Systems (IFS) sessions. The first one is how to introduce IFS and The Polyvagal Theory with a sandtray, the second is an IFSsandtray which displays working with two trays. One tray with figurines of the IFS concept of Self, and the other tray a with figurines of a current issue which the client is struggling with.

Chapter 15, **How to Use The Pro-Symptom Belief Cards with or without Miniatures** describes how to use the Pro-Symptom Belief Cards (PSBC) in the sandtray. Betty, utilizing the PSBC and how to access and heal Parts somatically and hypnotically while focusing on a core negative belief that accesses upsetting or traumatic childhood events.

Section Four: "Outcomes of Client's Healing Expeditions" shares the authentic success stories of clients who have healed from the therapeutic method of accessing the unconscious mind. Their experiences with IFSsandtray, Kalffian Sandplay, utilizing Internal Family Systems combined with Sensorimotor Psychotherapy through the Polyvagal Theory lens, and other techniques helped them in their healing from mental and sexual health issues. These individuals give testimonial to how they experienced skepticism to accepting and valuing their unconscious mind to heal them from the inside out.

Chapter 16, **Soul Reflections: Discovery of Self-Acceptance** describes how the body heals itself, as will the mind if given the right conditions. We revisit John and Billy who were labeled by professionals as sex addicts, only to find there was more to their psychological, mental, and sexual heath-presenting issues. Also, Jane shares a very touching story about her relationship with her partner David.

Chapter 17, **Client's Reflections of Their Self-Acceptance with In-Depth Therapy** includes stories from a few clients who wanted to share their experiences. These brave individuals describe, in their own words, what happened to them in our sessions far better than I could. Testimony includes stories from Grace and William, a couple who struggled with navigating the swinging lifestyle, Leona who is a member of the kink community tells her views of both sandplay and IFSsandtray, and finally a message from Cleopatra, a pseudonym named after her favorite miniature. Cleopatra suffered from complex childhood trauma and sang the praises of Sandplay.

Chapter 18, **The Conclusion: Beginner's Mind In Trusting the Process** focuses on the future of treating trauma with the unconscious in mind, with an understanding of the Polyvagal Theory, the Neurosequential Model of Therapeutics, the neuroscience behind Kalffian Sandplay, integration of somatic, Parts, clinical hypnosis, and more. This chapter points to a way forward in healing trauma.

Section One
Mapping Out the Journey

Introduction

1

Amazing Things Happen When You Trust the Process

In the year 2023, mass shootings, political upheaval, rampant opioid addiction, and countless other conditions leave people feeling unsafe and dysregulated. It's no wonder many are increasingly living with psychological trauma, attention deficit disorder, and sexual issues. Some of these issues include out of control sexual behavior (OCSB), which is also referred to as problematic sexual behavior, sexual dysfunctions, such as vaginismus or erectile disorders, and a large majority of these individuals living with sexual and non-sexual shame.

Many acknowledge the solution lies with the mental healthcare system and the mental healthcare professionals. Unfortunately, many current licensed professionals are still using outdated treatment methods and they don't even realize it. This textbook provides the latest up-to-date approaches in non-pathologizing treatments, based on the most recent thinking in the field of psychotherapy.

Practitioners still relying on the DSM-5-TR might consider OCSB and problematic sexual behavior as addictions. Those diagnosed with attention deficit disorder might be viewed as flawed. Most likely, these clients are not diseased but are suffering from dysregulated autonomic nervous systems (ANS) and trauma. Often, they've experienced early childhood mis-attunement resulting in the very issues for which they seek help.

Trauma affects everyone, frequently appearing as a mental health or sexual disorder. Unfortunately, there are still healthcare professionals who don't recognize trauma symptomology. Frequently trauma and complex trauma symptoms resemble anxiety, depression, shame, and many of the aforementioned sexual health issues. This book invites professionals to discover the

DOI: 10.4324/9781003388302-2

therapeutic power of the unconscious mind and play when treating all the above and more.

Many clinicians working with children accept the therapeutic power of play, but what about adults? Why is play left out when working therapeutically with them? Studies have shown that incorporating play into adult treatment has proven effective.

Play is an important social and cognitive activity, but it is often disregarded, and rarely incorporated into treatment for adults, especially for those suffering from sexual health disorders. At most its use is minimized, secondary only to outmoded forms of treatment. However, current thinking posits that, in the therapeutic environment, it can heal both children and adults. Dr. Stephen Porges, an expert in the field and author of the Polyvagal Theory, detailed his understanding in an article entitled "Play as a neural exercise." In the article, Dr. Porges defends the roots of play as a necessary link to the "evolution of a neural mechanism that enables mammals to shift between mobilized fight/flight and calm socially engaging states." I have found that incorporating Kalffian Sandplay and Internal Family Systems Sandtray (IFSsandtray, a method I developed in 2018) in therapy with adults can help unlock the inner tools to heal from within.

In fact, behaviors or other symptomology act as protection for the client. By focusing on destigmatizing such behaviors and rethinking them, I have laid the groundwork for a new approach to mental and sexual health issues in my therapeutic practice. I remove the barriers of shame and look at my clients in a more holistic, healing light.

The information contained within these pages is informed by neuroscience—to clarify how trauma sufferers have no control over their ANS. Throughout, I will show how the psychological or physical issues often are a result of the ANS engaging—within milliseconds—when a threat is *perceived*. Often this looks like a mental or sexual health "disorder" as the ANS will seek regulation, and self-soothing, ultimately causing individuals to experience chaotic behaviors and a range of emotions.

The body can—and frequently does—heal itself; the mind will do the same if given the proper conditions: a safe environment and a skillfully attuned therapist who can help clients access their inner psyche to utilize the healing power of the unconscious mind. In this milieu, the ANS will begin to enter a state known as ventral vagal, which can be described as calm, curious, and connected. It is only in this state where therapeutic change can happen.

This book presents integrated therapeutic modalities I have developed. These treatments have proved applicable to many adults with mental and sexual health issues. The applications of these therapies, including play, can apply to all seeking help. Throughout the text, we will see how others, not just those suffering from OCSB, ADD, and other mental and sexual issues, can benefit from the powerful healing properties. The principles covered within are valuable additions to any therapist's toolkit.

Throughout, I will explore how to identify the root of the problem, and how practitioners can facilitate healing in an empowering, intriguing, and soulful way. Many talk therapy techniques—like Cognitive Behavioral Therapy (CBT) and the standard modalities often covered in bachelor's and master's classes—may appear to alleviate symptoms (often temporarily), but never address the root of the issue, which remains deeply buried.

Understanding how the brain develops from the bottom up starting in infancy is one of the key principles I delve into in this book. The Neurosequential Model of Therapeutics (NMT) was designed by Dr. Bruce Perry and along with the research of Dr. Lorraine Freedle using the NMT in sandplay, changed my view of how people can heal.

The latest research and theories developed by other experts in the field of trauma, ADD, Shame, etc., Dr. Richard Schwartz, Dr. Jeffery Rediger, Dr. Stephen Porges, Deb Dana, Dr. Pat Ogden, Eric Erikson, and others are referenced to support my treatment approach. This approach will prove both timely and timeless, providing a framework for you, the professional, with various skill levels to stabilize, ground, and recognize. The effects of early attachment wounding as well as the dysregulated ANS's underlying most issues, and severe trauma can be complex and devastating. I have learned to trust an integrated approach, shown in the following chapters, in treating individuals. This assists them in discovering that they hold the very solutions necessary for their healing within themselves.

As complicated as the subject of trauma is, this integrated and systematic approach into the unconscious mind offers an accessible therapeutic method for healing that engages clients with deeply personal metaphor. This book also illustrates how symptoms of trauma are often mistaken as mental and sexual health disorders. The practice of the methods described herein is carefully laid out for professionals to work with clients through the non-pathologizing lenses of the Polyvagal Theory, The Neurosequential Model of Therapeutics, and metaphor.

Incorporating metaphor and imagery in your practice can help unlock the unconscious. To that end, I have designed "Pro-Symptom Belief Cards" (PSBC), based on common negative beliefs held by most clients. These beliefs, although they aren't actually true, were most likely learned before the age of five. Yes, before five; and many times, before four years of age. See Chapter 9, "Betty: Healing Early Childhood Trauma with the PSBC with IFS, and Sensorimotor" and Chapter 15, "How to Use the Pro-Symptom Belief Cards with or without Miniatures."

By shifting the focus away from such pathologizing terms as "sex addiction," the book addresses how treatment of these issues has rapidly advanced in the last five or so years. Throughout we will delve into the body/mind connection by looking at how the ANS instinctually protects the individual, often resembling mental and sexual health issues.

How we as professionals approach and view trauma, attention deficit disorder, shame, and the overall treatment of mental and sexual health issues must change. By incorporating our understanding of the ANS, and applying principles learned from neuroception (the five senses), we can access the unconscious, and thus find a new pathway to treatment.

While working with a client who experienced problematic sexual behavior, I had a question regarding that client's responses which could only be explained by neuroception. In response to my email about this observation Dr. Porges stated:

> Although I have never researched OCSB specifically, I speculate that OCSB is an attempt to regulate physiological state through sexual activity because engaging in sexual stimulation and orgasm allows them to move the autonomic state through sympathetic activation (sexual arousal) that would be followed by an autonomic calming (i.e., vagal surge) post orgasm. I would also speculate individuals who expressed OCSB would have a deficit in regulating physiological state through safe and trusting social interactions (e.g., via the social engagement system).
>
> (Personal communication, August 18, 2020)

The ANS perceives threats from the past, sending messages to the body, which reacts as if they are happening in the present moment. This explains the instinctive automatic engagement of the flight, fight, and submission defenses of that system's inherent trauma-related autonomic responses. The result is the appearance of mental and sexual health issues, such as OCSB, vaginismus, ejaculation issues, attention deficit, and much more.

Additionally, many clients who experience problematic sexual behavior suffer from loneliness because their behavior often isolates them from their partner and/or family. Indeed, it is the influences of loneliness, grief, and loss that can cause an individual to seek external means to regulate their physiology through acting out sexually. As evidenced in the work of Dr. Porges, the

Polyvagal Theory can aid in deconstructing grief, loss, or loneliness, which often disrupt our biological need to connect with others. See Chapter 11 and the case of Billy for an example of how loneliness led to shame and OCSB.

Like Billy, many clients hold core negative beliefs about themselves. In the 2020 book, *Cured: Strengthen Your Immune System and Heal Your Life*, Dr. Jeffery Rediger, states, "A more scientific term for it is your default mode network (DMN). The DMN is basically a collection of loosely connected regions of the brain, both older structures deep in the brain and newer ones in the cerebral cortex, which are activated, or light up, when you engage in certain categories of thinking. I say 'light up' because that's what it looks like on an fMRI—areas of the brain glow bright out of the silvery gray light when you blow on embers in a fire." This understanding led me to design the PSBC to access these belief patterns. These beliefs often stem from early childhood. See Chapters 9 and 15 for more on core negative beliefs and the PSBC.

The chapters within this book begin with an introduction to the ANS and the latest treatment modalities used in conjunction with accessing the unconscious, such as IFS, Sensorimotor Psychotherapy, Hypnosis, Sandtray, and Sandplay. The topic of DMN and the PSBC are covered in Chapters 8, 10, and 15. Stories from several individuals who undertook treatment provide needed insight into the inner workings of how to work with compassionate treatment methods.

Among the revelatory stories, I introduce you to a woman who was told by her gynecologist she would never have penetrative sex with a man, and how her time with me led to healing from this chronic condition in just 11 sessions.

This is a virtual guidebook for those who have been misled by the pathologizing of various sexual behaviors or mental health pathologizing diagnoses. This approach suggests an optimistic outlook that will enlighten you as a professional seeking more advanced measures in treating your clients, and expanding your "tool kit" as well as helping clients harness the unconscious mind to aid in healing.

Many doctors have utilized the acronym MUS (Medically Unexplained Symptoms) to describe what they can't elucidate. I will shed light on some of their potential sources. In a personal correspondence, Dr. Stephen Porges wrote, "The category of medically unexplained symptoms are, in general, features of dysautonomia. These would include irritable bowel syndrome, fibromyalgia, migraine, etc. They have the title of MUS because the medical profession cannot identify a causal influence/mechanism or an effective treatment. Polyvagal Theory suggests that MUS is the naturally occurring consequence of an ANS being in a chronic state of threat" (July 20, 2021).

To gain a more complete understanding of the polyvagal theory, see Chapter 4, "Innate Abilities to Navigate Difficult Terrain: Introduction to the Polyvagal Theory." In combination with a greater understanding of how trauma is held in the body (see Chapter 6, "Descending and Ascending: *Exploring Trauma: IFS & The Nervous System*" practitioners can gain a more complete, holistic understanding of their clients.

Those not familiar with the powerful IFS modality (and those already trained in IFS) will gain a new understanding of all human beings' physiological responses to emotions, referred to in IFS as "Parts." See Chapter 5, "Multiplicity: Introduction to Parts in Therapy." Practitioners will gain an understanding of how somatic experiences are locked in the body of the client and how Parts hold trauma in their metaphorical bodies.

Bessel van der Kolk, M.D. wrote the *New York Times* bestselling book, *The Body Keeps The Score: Brain, Mind, and Body in the Healing of Trauma* in 2014 where he wrote about IFS and Parts. He stated, "Each split-off part holds different memories, beliefs, and physical sensations; some hold shame, others the rage, some the pleasure and excitement, and another the intense loneliness …" Yes, Parts do hold the physical sensations and that is the very key needed to heal them. Parts holding the client's shame, anger, loneliness, and other emotions often resulting in behaviors seen in ADD, OCSB, and many other mental health and sexual disorders will be discussed throughout the pages contained within the following chapters.

Regrettably, to this day, far too many professionals are required to use the Diagnostic and Statistical Manual of Mental Disorders (DSM) to get paid by the client's health insurance provider. The result is the client believing something is wrong with them as they identify themselves as the diagnosis.

Something must change in the future and the future is now. It is *imperative* for professionals to be allowed to offer more thoughtful, non-pathologizing, and less stigmatizing answers to clients or patients. They must be allowed to trust in themselves and their own insights and has nothing to do with what the DSM classifies as illnesses (diagnoses), when in fact it is often the underlying trauma caused by early childhood upsetting experiences or trauma.

References

Porges, S., Personal communication about OCSB, August 18, 2020.

Porges, S., Personal communication about medically unexplained symptoms, July 20, 2021.

Porges, S. W., Play as a neural exercise: Insights from the Polyvagal theory. In S. W. Porges (Ed.), *Polyvagal safety: Attachment, communication, self-regulation*. W. W. Norton & Company, New York, NY, 2021 (pp. 61–65).

Rediger, J., *Cured: Strengthen your immune system and heal your life*. Flatiron Books, New York, NY, 2020 (p. 269).

van der Kolk, B., *The body keeps the score: Brain, mind, and body in the healing of trauma*. Penguin Books, New York, NY, 2014 (p. 284).

Cutting-Edge Psychotherapy Using Sand in Treatment

2

You may wonder, *what does sand have to do with sex therapy?* In my practice, I have found that using sand becomes one portal to a profound, mysterious place where therapeutic healing occurs, often spontaneously.

I have designed my psychotherapy office to offer a special place that brings about an *experiential milieu* for growth. In the center of my sandplay room stand two custom-made waterproof wooden trays. One important aspect of each tray is the blue interior covering both the base and sides. This provides the impression of depth, suggesting the ocean, or the vastness of the sky, which many associate with the unknown, the unconscious. The corners of the trays are linked together with dovetail joints; this technique, used in fine furniture, securely joins the wooden corners where one-piece interlocks with another. The trays are made to the exact dimensions of 28.5 in. by 19.5 in. by 2.75 in. The precise dimensions invite clients to view the entire tray without moving their heads. This becomes a critical feature in many therapy sessions when I later incorporate other useful modalities; *IFS* and *Sandtray,* Eye Movement Desensitization and Reprocessing (EMDR), Internal Family Systems (IFS), and Sensorimotor Psychotherapy.

Often during the initial consultation, I bring my clients into this area of my office. When they enter the room, I usually hear, "Wow! This is amazing!" I nod my head in agreement and begin to explain what they are observing. Usually, I hear them take a deep breath. This breath is critical when bodies and brains adjust to a new, visually stimulating environment. The autonomic nervous system responds within milliseconds to new things.

DOI: 10.4324/9781003388302-3

The surrounding walls are lined with shelving, and on those shelves stand hundreds of small figurines, most of them under four inches in height. At this point, I begin to speak, "Here is where you are most likely to do most of your therapy with me. Let me give you a little tour." They follow me further into the room. "This wall is all mythological," I wave my hand over the shelves from just below the ceiling to the floor. "Over here are all types of domestic and wild animals." When I turn the corner, I say, "Here are all the houses, things that go into them, including food, furniture, and over here are various types of vehicles; planes, boats, ambulances, buses ..."

Going around the room I show how the figurines are grouped by themes, for example, "This is the area for images of death, grief, and darker symbols. In this area are many figures made to represent emotions people may have. Here's one that is curled up in a ball." I pick it up and display it to them.

Often, I hear, "I bet you have everything here" My reply is, "Someday, you may want something I don't have, and I will try to locate it for you. I also have art supplies available where you can use your own creativity to make the symbol and take it home or leave it here." Many times, when people make their own symbols it's more personal and allows them to experience a sense of control or agency.

The search for a specialized miniature is more difficult than one would think. Once when someone asked me, "Do you have a golden goose?" I didn't at the time, but persistence paid off, and I found one on Etsy in Russia. Its home is now in the animal section, placed with other birds.

This elaborate setup allows a client to delve deeper into the world of their personal—as well as the collective—unconscious, trusting in a process where the "great unknown," the human psyche, is allowed to guide the journey to inner healing. The specifically designed tray also acts, to the same extent, as an emotional vessel for the psyche to work within its specified boundaries. The psyche requires the limits, so it won't overwhelm the client. The unconscious is the great unknown, filled with complexities and hidden treasures of wisdom. but it can also be overwhelming, so boundaries are important.

In traditional talk therapy, the unconscious is not the first consideration in the treatment of sexual issues. I have found that when the unconscious is accessed in a safe, secure, protected space, healing can happen instinctively and intuitively (Kalff, D. 2020). Transformation occurs when the unconscious is allowed to bubble up to the surface of conscious awareness. Working in the sand with multiple miniature figurines supports unconscious communication: nonverbally through symbols. The sand invites a person out of their conscious intellect into internal reflection; they create and witness something they often can't explain in words.

One function of the unconscious is to lay patterns down. Carl Jung would call these archetypes. In the book *Four Archetypes: Mother/Rebirth/Spirit/Trickster* which was translated by R.F.C. Hull, Jung (1992) wrote, "Just as all archetypes have positive, favorable, bright side that points upwards, so also they have one that points downwards, partly negative and unfavorable, partly chthonic, but for the rest merely neutral"(p. 104). Archetypes have the potential to be perceived as both positive and negative and can be found in literature, stories, myths, fairy tales, religions, and dreams and are often themes which represent the human experience. Jung's reference to chthonic, or underworld, relates directly to his belief in the collective unconscious. Common archetypes include the hero or heroine overcoming obstacles, poverty to wealth, and other themes where one rises above their challenges. In Kalffian sandplay the sandplayers may find themselves discovering their own obstacles or journey through some of these very archetypes.

When clients are selecting the figurines, often they don't know why they are drawn to or repelled by a miniature. Before anyone begins picking figurines, they are informed this may happen and each miniature has all the qualities of archetypes as mentioned above. Some individuals will gather all their miniatures at once using a basket before going over to place them in the tray while others select one at a time going from wall to tray numerous times. Placement of these very objects in the tray matters a great deal in sandplay, but in sandtray where a directive is used, not as much.

Each of these figurines may symbolize a variety of meanings, all at once, from majestic qualities the client doesn't recognize in themselves to forbidden secrets, or long-forgotten or repressed upsetting childhood events. Each sandplay client scans the figurines, connecting with each one that adds to their untold narrative. The figurines are placed in the tray; the client's story unfolds. This version of the story, told from a nonverbal place where the unbearable moves into consciousness in the tray and then outside, feels more endurable to many. The sand tray acts like a treasure map; it allows the viewer to search for the hidden riches of the unconscious territory. The client plays in the sand tray, the unconscious reveals some of its secrets.

This transformation through working in the sand is a process that often represents a shift in the unconsciously held turmoil that was too agonizing to know consciously. The figurines capture the unknown qualities carried in the shadows of the mind. For many sex therapy clients, these shadows may be illuminating and the key to their transformation.

References

Jung, C. G., *Four archetypes: Mother/rebirth/spirit/trickster*. Bollingen Series. Princeton University Press, USA, 1992 (Originally published 1959) (p. 104).

Kalff, D. M., *Sandplay: A psychotherapeutic approach to the psyche*. Translated by B. Matthews. Analytical Psychology Press, Oberlin, OH, 2020 (Original work published 1966).

What Path to Choose? The Difference

3

Sandtray and Sandplay

The above quotation is used by many professional Kalffian sandplay therapists who use sand and miniatures as a modality for treating individuals in therapy. It emphasizes the importance of using hands—a way to access deeply rooted traumas held by the body, mind, and implicit memory. Bonnie Badenoch in her book *Being a Brain-Wise Therapist: A Practical Guide to Interpersonal Neurobiology* wrote,

> Working in the sand invites the implicit world, home of our earliest attachment wounds, to take symbolic form. Sometimes it provides a road around defenses; often it lets preverbal pain emerge; sometimes it makes concrete the feelings that a person has had difficulty communicating; sometimes it externalizes and contains inner anguish that has been too powerful to call to consciousness in other ways. Grounded in the body, sandplay unfolds through limbic region and cortex, and spans both hemispheres; the symbolic world unfolds into words.
>
> (Badenoch, 2008)

Originally, I used Badenoch's words to show the reader how working with sand and miniatures opens the implicit world where trauma is held. Then I read it more closely and I noted how Badenoch identified sandplay and not sandtray as the specific modality to do this.

Whether a client is going to engage in sandtray or sandplay, the power of each is profound. This chapter will introduce the reader, and some clinicians who currently work with sand and miniatures in their therapeutic practices, what the differences are between Sandtray and Sandplay.

DOI: 10.4324/9781003388302-4

Too often, many individuals use the words sandplay and sandtray as if they were interchangeable, but they are not. Each is a separate modality. It is like identifying Sensorimotor Psychotherapy and Internal Family Systems and categorizing both as the same modality because each works with the sensations in the body. The clinicians who have studied each of the latter modalities would all identify each one as an entirely separate type of treatment method. Both require years of training to become proficient. The same is true for Sandtray and Sandplay.

I use both the sandtray and sandplay modalities in my therapy practice as well as sensorimotor and Internal Family Systems (IFS). I know there will be completely different outcomes depending on which of these modalities I use with the client and where he, she, or they are in their therapeutic work this will determine what modality I choose.

Sandtray

Sandtray often involves the therapist using prompts or suggestions to guide the client. Sandtray is often based on the modalities in which the therapist is trained, such as Cognitive Behavior (CBT), Eye Movement Desensitization Reprocessing (EMDR), Internal Family Systems (IFS), or any other method. This gives the clinician a lens through which they will assist the client to externalize an emotion or presenting issues, such as anxiety, depression, or anger. The therapist might say to the client, "Would you like to make a tray showing your anxiety?" or "Can you pick a miniature to represent the anger?"

Sandtray has not yet been standardized in terms of a unified understanding of its methods and competencies. I hold memberships in two separate sandtray organizations: the World Association of Sand Therapy Professionals (WASTP) and the International Association for Sandtray Therapy. Unfortunately, it appears they are working separately and not united.

In my clinical practice I use my training in IFS as a major lens in my sandtray work, but also combine it with Sensorimotor psychotherapy and often incorporate EMDR. IFS is an integral part of sandtray for me because of the concept of the multiplicity of the mind. Each emotion is considered valuable, often a protector, and helps the individual in some way. In the IFS comprehensive training, the clinician is taught how to work with these emotions, known and labeled as "Parts." Combining sensorimotor psychotherapy with IFS and a sandtray has been profound when working with Parts. Each Part has a body that can feel sensations somatically and can be accessed therapeutically. When this happens it often exposes a vulnerable Part that holds the trauma. All of this can be externalized in the tray and the vulnerable Part can be healed as well as the Part that was protecting it.

Even within the community of IFSsandtray practitioners, treatment varies greatly. Not all agree on the methodology and how it applies to sandtray. One group of certified IFS clinicians wrote an article with guidelines, outlining the use of sandtray, a nine-step process (Hodgdon et al., 2022). Other therapists, however, like myself, may not use this nine-step process, instead using sandtray in an entirely different way. Understanding the distinctions and recognizing the many variations, I created a website in 2018, www.IFSSandtray. com, to introduce my own method, IFS-sandtray. I follow the approved IFS model learned in the IFS trainings and incorporate both sensorimotor psychotherapy and EMDR.

Because of its flexibility and vast scope, sandtray offers each therapist the opportunity to choose the path and method that works right for them. This isn't a one-size-fits-all solution, but a methodology that provides a myriad of possibilities to enrich any therapist's tool kit.

Sandplay

When the word *sandplay* is used, it is most likely referring to Kalffian sandplay which was named so by Dora Kalff, the founder, who based sandplay on Jungian theory, Eastern philosophy, and play therapy she learned from Margaret Lowenfeld's World Technique. This is further explained later in this chapter.

Unlike sandtray, sandplay has been standardized and has been recognized internationally by the International Society of Sandplay Therapists (ISST). Many countries in the world follow the same process with their clients as any other Kalffian sandplay professional. This allows any sandplay client to enter therapy with any sandplay professional and the procedures and therapy will be similar. The ISST organization requires all sandplay professionals to undertake professional training, do their own personal process, engage in supervision with a certified teaching member, and write three major papers.

In Kalffian sandplay the therapist doesn't give a directive. Rather than prompt the client with a specific question or guiding thought, the therapist might ask something more general, such as "Would you like to use the sand today?" or "Would you like to make a tray today?" The clinician will not tell the client how to pick miniatures. The client is informed that there is no right or wrong way to make a sandplay picture.

It is suggested that the client might pick miniature figurines that seem to "come to them" or "figures that they are drawn to or even repelled by."

A Kalffian therapist will witness in silence the client's process in the sand. Should the client engage verbally with the clinician, the clinician will then respond accordingly. After the client stops placing the miniatures in the tray, the therapist will ask the client if it *feels* complete and might ask if they would like to share thoughts about the world they created. Today I had a client who made a sandplay tray and when I asked her if she wanted to share about the world, she said to me, "It's just so weird when you go around the room and pick things and you don't know what you are going to do with it." Many of my sandplay clients say similar things to me, as I did to my own sandplay therapist when I was healing through my own sandplay process.

Some sandplay therapists may include sandtray methods in their work; however, not all sandtray clinicians are trained in the process of Kalffian sandplay. The primary differences are explained in the below section.

Differences Between Kalffian Sandplay and Sandtray

Kalffian Sandplay

- Based on Jungian theory and concepts, Margaret Lowenfeld's World Technique, and Eastern philosophy
- Jungian concept of individuation is important
- Based on the work of Dora Kalff
- Nondirective
- Nonverbal
- Therapist witnesses silently
- Therapist holds "free and protected space"
- Delayed interpretations
- Unconscious focused
- Series of trays over a period of time
- Tray is a specific rectangular size (19.5" × 28.5" × 3")
- Personal in-depth sandplay process required from a credentialed therapist
- Formal international training and certification process
- Certification is internationally recognized

Sandtray

- Based on the theoretical lens of the therapist
- Often directed by the therapist
- Therapist may use interpretations
- Focus on developing insight

- Based on the training of the therapist
- Tray can be any size or shape
- Variation in the certification process
- Certification may or may not require personal sand work

Similarities of Kalffian Sandplay and Sandtray

- Use miniature figurines and sand
- Both are experiential methods
- Based on a trusting relationship between therapist and client

On December 27, 2021, *The Journal of Aggression, Maltreatment and Trauma* published an article titled, "Internal Family Systems (IFS) Therapy for Posttraumatic Stress Disorder (PTSD) among Survivors of Multiple Childhood Trauma: A Pilot Effectiveness Study." IFS, and its understanding of how the mind is made of multiple Parts, has heavily influenced this book. Throughout my practice, I have applied this theory to my sand practice, accessing the various Parts through the interplay with sand. Although the article itself and the research contained no mention of using sand in therapy, it explains how IFS is an effective tool used in the treatment of childhood trauma and the symptoms that come with it. These symptoms are typically depression, dissociation, somatization, shame, guilt, and even some of the negative core beliefs an individual may carry about themselves. Some of those beliefs are, "I am not good enough," "I am a failure," and many more.

The article reviews IFS concepts of mindfulness and multiplicity of the mind with subpersonalities. For example, the use of Parts or emotions, self-compassion, and the understanding "that each person has an inherent internal capacity for healing, the Self is our intuitive, core emotional and intellectual center" (p. 25). This study explores the effectiveness of IFS, an alternative treatment for PTSD. Within the article the authors write, "IFS is a comprehensive model of treatment, addressing all dimensions of the traumatic experience, including distorted thoughts and memories, traumatic affect, and physical sensations, from a mindful and compassionate perspective. IFS focuses on overwhelming affect and symptoms directly and early in treatment, minimizing the need for grounding strategies, resourcing, or safety stabilizing techniques" (p. 42).

The idea of not needing to establish stabilizing or grounding strategies, such as a safe space in eye movement desensitization reprocessing (EMDR), was one of the first concepts in IFS that surprised me when I was in the intensive IFS training. In these other modalities, I was taught that grounding the traumatized individual was essential. It is considered necessary in EMDR for the client to have a safe place and grounding experiences before the clinician makes any attempts in healing the traumatizing material the client holds within. Whereas in IFS the protective Parts will not allow the therapist to go deeper in treatment unless they give permission. This is taught in the first level of IFS training.

Many times, after an IFSsandtray session, the client feels relief from whatever emotion or issue they worked with that day. The client may say, "I had no idea my anger was actually trying to help me," or, "I didn't realize that my actions were my body and mind's way of trying to protect me."

Sandplay History

Dora Kalff (1904–1990) combined her knowledge of Margaret Lowenfeld's work with her own understanding of Jungian theory and Eastern contemplative practices. Her knowledge of Eastern philosophy, play therapy, and her Jungian training informed her "sandplay," her chosen name for the method. Below are the three roots of sandplay.

The Three Roots of Sandplay

Root One

The first root of Sandplay therapy as mentioned by Mitchell and Friedman (1999) was based on Kalff's training with child psychologist Margaret Lowenfeld (1890–1973). After attending a lecture given by Margaret Lowenfeld in 1954, Kalff discussed with Carl Jung her thoughts on going to England to study with Lowenfeld. Jung recalled being impressed by Lowenfeld years earlier in 1937 after she had presented at a conference he had attended (p. 49).

According to Mitchell and Freidman (1999) Margaret Lowenfeld spoke only English early in her life and spent summers with her cousins who only spoke German. This experience was instrumental in her interest in nonverbal communication and left her skeptical of verbal language as the only method of communication (pp. 5–7). This was a major part of the formulation of her work helping children through expressive means. The children could be "heard" without any use of verbal language.

In 1928, Lowenfeld opened the Children's Clinic for the Treatment and Study of Nervous and Difficult Children. Tatum (2018) wrote that Lowenfeld's clinic was a wonderful, safe environment for children to undergo treatment. They were given access to two zinc trays, one filled with water, another with sand, and miniatures where the children made "worlds." Her method became known as "The World Technique" (pp. 70–71). Lowenfeld realized the importance of the use of these zinc trays in her treatment, containing either dry or wet sand. Lowenfeld innately understood how this was fundamental in the healing of her clients. The use of toys, sand, and water was also fundamental to Kalff, who later recognized a sequential patterning in the sandplay work of her clients.

Around the time Lowenfeld opened her clinic, she read an original work by the prolific author, H. G. Wells (1866–1946). Perhaps one of his least-known works, it was an account of how he played with his sons. This can be found in his book *Floor Games, A Father's Account of Play and Its Legacy of Healing*. Turner (2004) writes that Wells wrote this book for parents to read so they could become better parents (p. 100). Mitchell and Friedman (1999) emphasize Well's belief that children's play would ultimately allow them to become creative and healthy individuals (p. 2). Dora Kalff, encouraged by Carl Jung, went on to study at Margaret Lowenfeld's clinic for one year in 1956. She was mentored that year by Michael Fordham, the first Jungian child therapist in London. She also studied with D. W. Winnicott.

Root Two

The second root of sandplay comes by way of Kalff's Jungian training and her analysis with Carl Jung's wife, Emma Jung. According to Mitchell and Friedman (1999) it was in therapy with Emma that Kalff discussed having dreams of being in Tibet. Another dream occurred on the night of Carl Jung's death. In that dream she was having dinner with Jung and in the middle of the table was a mound of rice. Jung pointed to the rice and indicated to Kalff she should continue her exploration of the East (pp. 50–51). This became the beginning of the journey Kalff embraced with passion.

Root Three

The third root of sandplay was based on Kalff's study and practice of Eastern philosophies. She possessed an inner wisdom, compassion, and a love for the East. Mitchell and Friedman (1999) write, "Kalff's Asian studies greatly impacted her work which bridged both Eastern and Western cultures. During the time of the invasion of Tibet, Kalff opened her home to a Tibetan lama evacuee. Kalff was also greatly influenced by the Zen Buddhist scholar, D. Suzuki, who invited her to Japan where she later taught sandplay. It was from their meetings that Kalff realized the importance of delaying the interpretation of the work of her clients, seeking wisdom, and redirecting questions back to the person so they could reflect on what the questions might mean" (pp. 50–52).

Jung (1963) writes about his own life challenges, including an early trauma when his mother was hospitalized (p. 8). Jung further wrote about the ongoing challenges of having two personalities, number one, and number two. The number one personality was dealing with the external world whereas the number two personality inhabited his inner world. These two personalities conflicted with each other; number one caused his depression while in number two he found great comfort (p. 80). It is through personality two that we begin to understand Jung and his connection to sandplay. This personality, attracted to symbols and prone to contemplate the unknown, questioned dogma. Jung wrote in 1989 about how upsetting the separation from Freud had been to him because he lost many friends and acquaintances (p. 167).

Jung experienced tremendous isolation when he and Freud dissolved their relationship; Jung's life became chaotic. Mitchell and Friedman write about this period, and how he alleviated some of the pain by building earth and stones structures on the lakeshore (p. 50). Jung (1963) described how it was through these difficulties that he became stronger and noted if he hadn't experienced the traumas of the outside world, he never would have known his inner world where he developed "a kinship with all things" (p. 359).

Although in sandtray, with its prompts, directives, and various modality lenses, things may seem like sandplay with both using a tray of sand, miniatures, and sometimes water, but they provide different insights into the nature of trauma and healing. I use both modalities in my therapeutic work because I believe they lead to different outcomes. Sandtray is powerful; it works with aspects of the individual's persona or when they feel stuck with a particular issue or problem. These clients can externalize the emotions or issues by selecting specific miniatures and placing them in the tray.

Sandplay is an in-depth therapeutic process where many individuals with complex trauma and or severe PTSD can heal without ever having to relive the trauma. This draws on the right hemisphere of the brain, where human beings are creative and can solve solutions by thinking in metaphor. The figurines, which contain both positive and negative attributes, multilayered in meaning, allow the right hemisphere to creatively solve the problem. This is usually a result of a series of trays where the client's right hemisphere is allowed to do what the left hemisphere cannot because it is logical, linear, and mathematical I love it when I have an issue and I can "sleep on it" and wake up with the answer. That is the role of the right hemisphere in creatively solving problems. Sandplay is like seeing a dream before you.

Basically, Kalffian Sandplay is an unguided approach to accessing the unconscious with play. Sandtray, by contrast, relies on tools the therapist provides with guided prompts and is directive.

References

Badenoch, B., *Being a brain-wise therapist: A practice guide to interpersonal neurobiology.* W.W. Norton, New York, NY, 2008 (p. 220).

Hodgdon, H. B., Anderson, F. G., Southwell, E., Hrubec, W., & Schwartz, R., "Internal family systems (IFS) therapy for posttraumatic stress disorder (PTSD) among survivors of multiple childhood trauma: A pilot effectiveness study," *Journal of Aggression, Maltreatment & Trauma*, 2022, pp. 22–43. https://doi.org/10.1080/10926771.2021.2013375

Jung, C. G., *Memories, dreams, reflections.* Random House, New York, NY, 1989 (Original work published 1963).

Mitchell, H., & Friedman, R., *Sandplay past, present, & future.* Routledge, London, 1999 (Original work published 1994).

Tatum, J., "The Green Apron: The pioneering work of Margaret Lowenfeld," *The Journal of Sandplay Therapy*, 27(1), 2018, pp. 69–74.

Turner, B., *H.G. Wells' floor games a Father's account of play and its legacy of healing.* Temenos Press, Cloverdale, CA, 2004 (Original work published 1911).

Innate Abilities to Navigate Difficult Terrain

4

Introduction to the Polyvagal Theory

Anxiety, depression, guilt, shame, and other uncomfortable emotions aren't all in our heads. We carry them around on our bodies, like battle scars. We've all heard the expression "they wear their emotions on their sleeve," dismissing these people as being over-emotional, perhaps even unstable. What if we all wear our emotions not only on our sleeves, but on our entire body, from morning to night, our emotional lives plastered large across our backs, legs, chest, and arms? In my sessions with John, a pseudonym, I learned to pay close attention to this.

He initially contacted me by email, and his message suggested that he was very invested in comprehending what he was doing and why. In his original email to me, he wrote, "I put myself before my daughter and family, and have been going to massage parlors to receive arousing euphoric states and sometimes actually letting the massage person masturbate me. I also feel like my life has been extremely self-centered and selfish, as a result I am not having the types of loving, and depth filled relationships I want to have in life." I was impressed with this statement; he already had some understanding of his inner world. It felt like he was ready to grow.

The moment I read "euphoric states," my thoughts turned to his autonomic nervous system (ANS). In this distressing email, I recognized how John obviously was not enjoying his visits to massage parlors; his internal shame

DOI: 10.4324/9781003388302-5

was beating him up. Many of my clients experience a disconnect between their external behaviors and their internal emotional states. John's mismatch spoke volumes to me because I have worked with numerous individuals struggling with similar predicaments. His emotional agony, sorrow, heartache, and discomfort frequenting massage parlors suggested to me that he was experiencing problematic out of control sexual behavior (OCSB). His actions and behaviors were meant to cause an internal shift or response and they had great negative consequences. These misguided attempts to regulate his internal state were instead causing him pain and shame. Contacting me through his email represented a huge leap and demonstrated his willingness to begin his next stage of growth.

It was late afternoon on a cool, brisk November day. I opened the door, eager to see John, who by now I'd been working with just about every other week, for a total of seven sessions at that point. On that day he wasn't smiling, as was his custom. Tall and tousled, he looked a bit worse for wear after a day of working outdoors. Immediately I could see he was in turmoil. He lumbered heavily into the room, dragging his feet. His shoulders slouched forward, and his hair was rather messy because he had just come from his job, where he worked all day outdoors. Although I find the crisp fall air invigorating, I could see that it had little impact on him. Instead, he looked exhausted and defeated. Still dressed in his work attire, which included a heavy-weight winter jacket with the company logo emblazoned on the upper-left chest. A large sweat stain on his sweatshirt across the heart area belied a day of hard work. His dungarees appeared gently worn, perhaps like something he would wear if visiting with an old friend. Despite the somewhat frayed and tattered look of his attire, he gave the impression of someone comfortable in his clothing and in his own skin.

John walked over to the sofa, collapsed into the middle seat, taking the weight off his feet, and parked himself. I noticed how his spine curved outward, not supporting the lumbar area of his back. He threw his head and shoulders backward; I was a tad worried since his head was only being held up by the semi-attached back cushions of the couch. He was almost in a prone position, both of his legs were stretched forward, grazing the coffee table in front of him. His heels were touching the floor, and his toes pointed straight up in the air. He kept tugging at his jeans around the knees, displaying his discomfort. Finally, he made eye contact with me and drew in a long, deep breath. My body and mind knew something was wrong immediately. What could this possibly mean?

I began, "It's been two weeks since I last saw you. How's it going?"

"My wife and I have been really connecting in the last two weeks. Sex has been amazing, and we've been able to talk about a lot of different things."

I certainly hadn't thought he would say something like that. I wondered how his body and movements could be so out of alignment with what he just told me—I prompted him for more information. "John, tell me more."

"I had a great couple of weeks. Our three-year-old daughter hasn't been sleeping or going to bed till way past 10 o'clock. I never knew how a young child could rule the roost." His body shifted, and he held his head down, no longer making eye contact. He paused for a few seconds, then slowly added in a much sadder tone, "I feel so guilt-ridden and shameful. I can't believe what I've done."

Ah, I thought to myself, the mismatch had arrived; awareness and John's authenticity were entering the session. When he opened up to me about these emotions, I was flooded with compassion and felt a warm feeling in my own body. I rely on my own internal observations and resultant reactions to gauge the well-being of my clients.

John, like so many others suffering from dysregulated ANS, described to me symptoms like anxiety, depression, guilt, shame, and other uncomfortable emotions. These symptoms are indications or warning signs stemming from the ANS showing dysregulation. The body has developed its own built-in defense system for when it senses something is wrong in the outside world, resulting in instantaneous physiological and psychological shifts.

The ANS operates below the level of conscious awareness (subcortical brain), ascertaining in milliseconds whether situations are dangerous or innocuous. Thank goodness for this, or saber-toothed tigers would have eaten us long ago! This adaptation in the human body is wired to sense the slightest hint or cue of danger or threat. When you consider that the ANS is an integral aspect of the human body that interacts with every other system, including organs, it's no wonder that the medical field has an acronym called, MUS or medically unexplained symptoms.

The ANS gets wired in early childhood, taking in external cues from the environment, caregivers, and other sources. If the circumstances for children are consistently nurturing, nonviolent, and secure, and reliable caretakers meet their needs, the young child will learn how to self-soothe very early in life and maintain and grow this ability. This flexible resilience is a highly coveted skill for all human adults. However, if these childhood conditions and milieus are precarious, unstable, violent, unpredictable, and insecure, that person will not be able to reliably alleviate their stress levels or reliably regulate their ANS in adulthood. John had explained in an earlier session that his own childhood had been tumultuous, with an alcoholic father and a chaotic household. This can have grave consequences.

The ANS's hypersensitivity is ultimately a protector of the body. The ANS has patterns for interpreting the present circumstances or situations. These patterns are often replications of what happened in childhood. In families where abuse and neglect are present (i.e., unsafe families, especially if the original caregivers themselves were not safe, sound, and trustworthy), these patterns get hardwired into the developing person's ANS. Early childhood experiences are locked in a compartment of the mind that can later be triggered, often resulting in a felt sense of danger for the person. The human being is not consciously aware of the cues of danger that were once known by the inner child metaphorically trapped in time. The cues of danger that awaken this inner child are sensed by the ANS, which responds instantaneously.

Peril or cues of threat to the inner world can be simple, an expression on a stranger's face or even a perceived threat heard in a benign sound, which can bring a jolt to the nervous system. For example, the simple sound of footsteps coming up a staircase can be the trigger to the inner child, it may be an all-encompassing sound to the nervous system, an unconscious reminder of a horrifying early childhood experience. These childhood occurrences become a baseline for numerous individuals who never speak a word of their abuse. Many times, I hear these individuals say to me, "I didn't have that bad of a childhood. I know many other people who suffered bad situations; they had it tougher than me." This denial can sound rational, and it keeps the terror locked in place. This is where unconscious processing work, achieved through sandplay, can really help unlock what is hidden so that it may be seen and healed.

Adults react to this terror in ways that may go against their values and beliefs because human bodies automatically respond to perceived dangerous situations. We have the ANS to thank for this. The term *out of control behavior* refers to just one of countless behavioral patterns, actions, and adaptations made to regulate or manage feelings of distress the ANS produces. Too many people experience this and can't believe how the ANS can be so powerful.

In addition, the ANS can also have an impact on the human sexual response system sometimes appearing to be sexual behaviors that the client feels are out of control. The polyvagal theory supports a non-pathological approach to healing these matters. Rather than working to suppress or obliterate the behavior, we can help the ANS become more flexible, resilient, and self-regulated. In other words, the polyvagal theory understands many presenting issues, the body essentially responding to cues of danger, either from the past or the present situation. Because humans are sexual beings, any reactions to indications of danger may present in the body, a variety of sex-related disorders including, vaginismus, erectile disorders, OCSB, and other sexual concerns.

OCSB typically develops to calm a dysregulated ANS; however, OCSB no longer must carry shame, guilt, or a label of addiction. OCSB is one of the most controversial topics in sex therapy. Currently, some call it "sex addiction," which is a deeply pathologizing label to those who struggle with a dysregulated ANS that is neuroception (another word for the five senses) sensing danger. In an effort to calm the ANS, these individuals may engage in behaviors that lead to orgasm to bring the natural chemicals of epinephrine, endorphins, serotonin, oxytocin, dopamine, and other endogenous (naturally occurring) drugs to momentarily calm the nervous system automatically. The release of these chemicals can create feelings of pleasure resulting in a temporary state of calmness known as ventral vagal.

Unfortunately, this enjoyable experience quickly fades once the individual becomes consciously aware of the OCSB behavior in which they engaged. That could be anything, such as looking at sexual imagery, going to a massage parlor, sex worker, or something else. At that moment the ANS will go into an immobilized state. This state is called the dorsal vagal state where individuals experience disconnection with themselves and others. This is discussed further in Chapter 6, Descending and Ascending: Exploring *Trauma: IFS & The Nervous System*.

When the ANS is in an immobilized state and the individual who uses sex to regulate often experiences shame as a rebound feeling. This contributes to the backlash—the shame creates a physical reaction that is tied to regret, causing the person to feel horrible about himself due to knowing he just performed the very behavior he wants to stop. This is often what creates the cycle some label as an addiction. It is not an addiction, but rather a physiological attempt in regulating the ANS.

To think about this a little differently, imagine a person who struggles with an entirely different circumstance—for example, asthma. When the inability to take a deep breath triggers an ANS response, the person feels panic. So, they use their inhaler to quell the panic and take that deep breath. This seems like a legitimate response. What if the person with asthma did this every two minutes for the entire day? This may evoke some negative responses from family and friends. The person might then feel embarrassed and ashamed simply because they wanted to quell panic or regulate their body's distress. This might cause them to hide their inhaler use or, even worse, withdraw entirely to avoid judgmental looks. This could become a negative cycle in their life, all because they wanted to feel calm and be able to breathe.

This analogy may be imperfect; we understand that asthma is, of course, entirely different from OCSB. However, the bodily reactions are basically the same. The ANS is in charge while the individual is struggling with an internal sense of panic, alarm, or even dread. Somatic therapies are specifi-cally designed to help clients reorganize their ANS and help them live more freely than they ever have before.

All of this came into play in this session with John. As I observed him physi-cally from the moment, he entered the room. His hunched-over body, the emotional disconnection, and his tugging at his jeans. His description of feel-ing symptoms of anxiety, depression, guilt, and shame. I knew this was the day to engage John in an exercise and learn about his own ANS.

"John, I would like to do an art project with you that should help you understand you own autonomic nervous system. I have done it myself and think this will help explain so much to you. We will cover the three basic states of the ANS, ventral vagal or when you experience calmness, sympa-thetic when you feel a lot of energy, and dorsal vagal when you feel depressed or have no energy. Is that something you might want to try today?"

"Okay, it sounds like it might be helpful, so I am all in."

The art project was based on one I learned on the first weekend of training I did in 2018 on The Polyvagal Theory with Deb Dana in Kennebunkport, Maine. It is also found in her book, *The Polyvagal Theory in Therapy: Engaging the Rhythm of Regulation* in the worksheet pages found on page 217 labeled, "The Personal Profile Map." While in training I did the art project, found it immensely helpful, and I began using it with all my clients right away. She lays out the foundation for this by using a ladder to describe how the ANS moves upwards and downwards.

There are three basic stations on this ladder: the top, middle, and bottom. In each area the individual will have a different view of themselves, how they perceive others, and how they will behave, depending on their place on the metaphorical ladder. The client draws pictures representing these three states. By doing this, the client can gain a better understanding of how they internally relate to each state, and helps them recognize how they see the world differently, depending on the state of their own ANS at any given time.

With this exercise, the client uses his own language to describe his feelings. John could say what he felt worked best for him; he didn't have to use the scientific language of ventral, sympathetic, and dorsal. He was able to draw a picture of what it felt like to be in that state, and then write down words to describe how he felt, and finally, he could fill in the blank of the following two sentences: "The world is _____ and I am _____ when I am at the top, middle or bottom of the ladder."

At the top of the ladder John called this "Bliss;" this was when he was his calmest and most centered. He listed the following activities, describing his personal state of Bliss: going to the beach, listening to the ocean, being with friends, shopping, and watching the New England Patriots win against a rival team. When asked how he saw the world, he said, "The world is safe, and I am happy." He drew a stick figure with a happy face.

In the middle of John's ladder, he called this "Despair." He listed the following in this category: "very angry, my body is tense; I yell, and I am opinionated; I want to be heard and respected; I have anxiety, and fear. The world is difficult, and I am crazy." He drew a stick figure with an anxious face and lines coming out of its head.

At the bottom of the ladder John called this "Helpless" and he described this, "not having any words, being depressed, sleeping, lying down, checked out, and not able to talk," he said. "The world is unbearable, and I am depressed." He drew a stick figure lying on its side in a bed.

He then said, "I now know I was really depressed and upset. I was at the bottom of the ladder. I didn't feel I could even begin to talk to Sophia even though I realize now I should have. That is the worst feeling and I hate myself for hurting her. I never wanted to hurt her. I just don't get why I even went. When I am feeling 'Helpless' I am completely shut down; I feel so shameful. It's a vicious cycle."

We discussed his current cycle where he would feel helpless and shut down after experiencing anxiety, anger, and fear. John didn't know how to soothe himself when he experienced these difficult emotions. This is typical of many individuals not just individuals with OCSB. Often those who had early childhoods like John who didn't learn to self-soothe in early childhood, and I explained that to him.

When I did this same exercise in the training, Deb taught the participants how to change their own cycles. I applied the same principles with John. Before we started, I told John we would start in the middle of the ladder followed by the lower section where I would suggest new ways of breaking his current cycle of regulating through sex. The reason to start in the middle of the ladder is because the individual's ANS may become sympathetically aroused when thinking about how they are triggered in that state. Once the middle is completed, the therapist has the client go to the bottom of the Personal Profile Map, dorsal vagal. Again, the individual can begin to experience that state while they are focusing on mapping their ANS.

Once that is completed, the therapist suggests physical ways to re-engage the client's body. First by simply making small movements, such as moving the head, the arms, etc. Deb informed all the clinicians in the room to always do what they are asking the client to do. I began making the same movements as John. Within moments he began to make bigger movements and was sitting up straighter on the sofa and looking me in the eyes.

The next step is to have the client move into a sympathetic state by learning new techniques. This time John and I discussed what he could do to mobilize or regulate differently than he had in the past cycle. A discussion ensued and John learned the benefits of engaging in activities that used his body, such as going for a walk or run, yoga, art, or training his dog. Sometimes, I will ask the client to engage in ten jumping jacks with me to show them how the body feels differently after moving. It works!

Finally, John and I mapped his blissful state of ventral vagal. He was now sitting up, looked calm, and said, "I get it now! The autonomic nervous system has a lot to do with sex, and it's so critical to understand." I nodded and smiled, appreciating that his therapy was helping him create greater awareness of the body-mind connection. John held eye contact with me and stood up from his seat. He said, "I am filled with hope along with a new understanding of the ANS and my OSCB."

"John, before you go, I would like for you to watch a few videos and read a little bit more about the Polyvagal Theory for homework, to have a more complete understanding of it, would you be interested in that?"

"Yes, absolutely," he said. "I would love that. Do you think I can watch it with my wife Sophia?"

"I think that would be perfect and so helpful for both of you." I wrote down the information for the Polyvagal Institute's website, www.polyvagalinstitute.com, where he and his wife could find videos and articles that explained the process more fully. I recommend these videos to all my clients because they provide a more in-depth explanation than we can possibly cover in one session. Also, by sharing them with their partner, both individuals can reframe the OCSB as dysregulation of the ANS rather than thinking of it as an addiction. John had taken great strides in that session, coming to a better understanding of how his state of mind could impact his decision making.

One thing I wanted to address before I close this chapter—a statement John made while he was mapping his system: "Oh, now I really get it. When I am at the top of my ladder in 'Bliss' I am feeling fabulous and have had no desire to go to the massage parlor. It's when I feel I am slipping into 'Despair' due to anxiety, work stressors or other hassles that I notice feeling I can't take it anymore, I *found myself* at the massage parlor."

As a clinician, when a client says they "found themselves" anywhere, it may feel as if they're relinquishing responsibility. I once believed that too, but since incorporating the non-pathologizing lenses of Polyvagal Theory and The Neurosequential Model of Therapeutics (NMT), Internal Family Systems (IFS), and the somatic work learned while studying Sensorimotor Psychotherapy, I no longer believe OCSB is an addiction cycle, but rather a cycle of trying to regulate a dysregulated ANS. Each modality listed above is extremely powerful by itself, but when combined and utilized collectively they are influential in creating a non-pathologizing lens in treatment.

NMT informs clinicians on how the brain develops from the brainstem, up to the midbrain, to the limbic system, and finally the cortex. It integrates neurodevelopment with what happened to an individual as a child who experienced upsetting events, mis-attunement, or trauma often resulting in difficulties in adulthood, such as OCSB and other DSM diagnoses.

IFS teaches therapists to see emotions through a unique lens, one where each emotion serves the system in an effort to protect a person. The concept of Self, which has qualities of calmness, curiosity, clarity, compassion, confidence, courage, creativity, and connectedness—all qualities found in the ventral vagal state. In addition, proactive emotions in IFS are called Managers, reactive ones known as Firefighters which can be thought of as the sympathetic state of the Polyvagal Theory (we will discuss this in more detail in Chapter 5).

Finally, Sensorimotor Psychotherapy teaches us that trauma is often trapped in the body somatically and indicates a method to follow the physical sensations in healing. Ultimately, we all wear our emotions on our sleeves and in our entire body, from morning to night, our emotional lives broadcasted by our very own physiques.

Reference

Dana, D., *The polyvagal theory in therapy: Engaging in the rhythm of regulation.* W. W. Norton & Company, Inc., New York, NY, 2018.

Multiplicity

5

Introduction to Parts in Therapy

They come to me anxious for relief, eager to find the way out from their problems, to encounter something that will help them heal. They've talked and talked, but they still end up right where they began. As a psychotherapist I have always sought out the latest innovative approaches in healing my clients, resulting in undertaking numerous trainings. In this chapter, I will discuss two of the various models of psychotherapy I have incorporated into my practice: Internal Family Systems (IFS), and Integrative Neuro Linguistic Programming (INLP). I incorporated IFS into my practice approximately thirteen years ago and within the last year INLP. I find both useful tools in my psychological tool kit. Both approaches are patient-driven, heal and resolve inner conflicts due to polarizations, as well as quelling the warring battle between two conflicting Parts.

Each modality operates on the concept that the personality comprises many thoughts and emotions, called "Parts." We frequently use a simplified example to explain parts, "A Part of me wants to do X and another Part of me doesn't." The "X" can signify any struggle or polarization an individual may have which is causing them to feel stuck and not moving forward with positive actions or healing. Examples include smoking, drug, or substance use, out of control sexual behavior (OCSB), erectile difficulties, or even vaginismus, which makes sexual penetration difficult or challenging, as well as other sexual issues.

In June 2015, Disney/Pixar released a fantastic movie called *Inside Out* which many IFS therapists to this day recommend to their clients, a fun,

DOI: 10.4324/9781003388302-6

wonderfully informative visualization of Parts held within a person's system. Fortunately, this movie does not overwhelm viewers the concept of Parts having their own Parts.

Internal Family Systems (IFS)

IFS was developed by Dr. Richard Schwartz in the 1980s. Trained in family therapy, Schwartz, at that time, was working with a specific population of clients who had eating disorders; many were bulimic. As a family therapist, Schwartz felt what was happening with his clients was a sequence of events or interactions, like what is found in a family system. He noticed these clients discussed how Parts of themselves caused them to engage in such behaviors. Schwartz first thought those clients might have been displaying Multiple Personality Disorder (MPD), until he realized he, too, had similar judgments about food. Furthermore, his own beliefs and thoughts about food were as intense as those of the clients he was treating. Dr. Schwartz became curious and wanted to understand more about what was happening with these individuals. He began to experiment with a new form of therapy, working with these individuals and helping them get to know their Parts.

I admired how IFS never uses pathologizing language to describe or box individuals into a diagnosis. Often—when I collaborate with therapists who are not familiar with the IFS model or Parts language—I literally discover a Part of myself that cringes when I hear a client being described as having an illness or personality disorder, such as borderline personality disorder (BPD). Those therapists might say something like, "he/she/they are 'a borderline.'" IFS has reframed how I, and many clinicians, view human beings, not their diagnoses, but rather seeing these individuals are made up of a variety of Parts. When a client presents with traits of the above-mentioned diagnosis (BPD), IFS reframes that to a client exhibiting extreme Parts. Often the person displaying extreme Parts experienced early childhood trauma or attachment wounds which were not emotionally or physically safe. Also, I want to make it clear, not all individuals who have been raised in emotionally or physically unsafe environments will have extreme Parts.

I would like to elaborate further on many aspects of IFS and will keep it simplified. With scores of books, articles, and YouTube videos available, anyone can access this information. Basically, IFS consists of three major components to comprehend: Self, Protectors (comprised of Managers and Firefighters), and Exiles—which are the Parts that hold the original wound, are stuck in time, and are the age of the inner wounded child. Frequently, protectors are not much older than a juvenile.

Self

Self is *not* considered a Part. It is *a state of being* where the body and mind are congruent and harmonious, where individuals can access mindfulness. Some liken this to a person's essence, and I consider it our "soul energy." While in this state, the autonomic nervous system is regulated, and the individual can focus, solve problems more easily with composure, and experience a sense of serenity, stillness, and tranquility. When human beings are in Self, their physiology shifts and is in the resilient state of "flow" seen in The Survive/ Thrive Spiral in chapter six.

Dr. Frank Anderson, a lead trainer and consultant for the IFS Institute, describes Self in his book, *Transcending Trauma: Healing Complex PTSD with Internal Family Systems Therapy* (2021), defining it: "An innate presence in each of us that promotes balance, harmony, and nonjudgmental qualities (curiosity, caring, creativity, courage, calm, connectedness, clarity, and compassion). The Self is a state of being that can neither be created nor destroyed" (pp. 7–8). All individuals have Self, and some individuals describe this when they are in their highest spiritual state. This is felt internally when they connect to their higher power, and resulting in them feeling peaceful, diplomatic, able to enjoy humor, be playful, and see other points of view without judgment.

Schwartz (2021) writes about Self, "when you experience Self, you naturally feel more connected to humanity in general, and also to something larger and more encompassing—the Earth, the universe, the big SELF, or whatever your experience of this is" (p. 99).

Protectors: Managers and Firefighters

Protectors are Parts that have taken on the role of protecting the system from extreme feelings which could overwhelm the person. Protectors are usually reactions to emotional triggers and often stem from our childhood wounds. These wounds are exiles in IFS (I'll elaborate further later in this chapter).

Managers

Manager Parts are diligent in making sure people present themselves well in life to others. I found Dr. Anderson's definition helpful in describing managers' "preventive parts," writing, "[preventive parts are] One of the two protective parts. The manager's goal is to keep exiled parts hidden by making sure the wound never gets activated. Manager types include conflict-avoidant, intellectual, obsession, worrying, and hardworking parts" (pp. 7–8). In addition, manager Parts are Protectors who try to keep a person in control of a situation and work to control the environment. Managers are very diligent at making a person look and act their best, so they won't be criticized or judged by another person.

Firefighters

Often individuals find themselves behaving in ways they would love to stop and find it difficult to end behaviors they dislike. Often this is typical of individuals who present with OCSB. I also see individuals struggling with other physical concerns, vaginismus, early or delayed ejaculation, difficulty maintaining erections, and a few other sexual issues. Every single one of these clients wants relief. I have noticed how the Parts will somaticize or physicalize in the client's body. Parts also have their own internal bodies, which can be tracked to the original wound held by an exile, and these Parts can present themselves physically as one or more of the sexual issues I have listed above.

I realized when many, if not all, of my clients, carry negative beliefs about themselves. These undesirable, adverse, and destructive thoughts have a direct connection to how and why the body, mind, and Parts react and behave. In the first session, I try to find out what unconstructive and harmful convictions each person carries. Usually, everyone has at least one, and usually five or more. I have come to understand that these beliefs are held by the Protectors, often a Firefighter.

In his book, *Cured: The Life-Changing Science of Spontaneous Healing*, Dr. Jeffrey Rediger (2020) calls these "limiting beliefs." He wrote, "It's undeniable that we all have foundational, core beliefs that we aren't aware of, that could be determining our capacity to heal. But how do we identify and then unravel beliefs that may be limiting or even damaging?" (p. 252) This limiting belief is often a Firefighter, trying to help yet unable to because it is reacting to an already triggered exile and is trying desperately not to become overwhelmed by the pain of the original wound. Dr. Rediger's research found limiting beliefs are held within the structure of the brain, calling this, "Default Mode Network (DMN)." He wrote, "The DMN is basically a collection of loosely connected regions of the brain, both older structures deep in the brain and newer ones in the cerebral cortex, which are activated, or light up, when you engage in certain categories of thinking" (p. 269).

Daniel J. Siegel, MD, a clinical professor of psychiatry authored the 2018 book titled, *Aware: The Science and Practice of Presence* he also discussed the DMN. He wrote, "Arising from the brain stem's first mapping of the body's signals, and then the limbic region's weaving together of a sense of emotion, motivation, evaluation, memory, and attachment, we then move up to the cortex. The new cortex, or mammalian or neocortex, grew in our mammalian evolution… This prefrontal cortex is a major integrative hub of the brain, linking cortex, limbic, brain stem, somatic, and even social flows of energy and information to each other" (p. 133).

This information helped me to understand emotions of anger or rage and others which are protective Parts in the IFS modality. The firefighting Parts involved issues around food including anorexia or bulimia. Other behaviors might include addiction to drugs, overwork, spacing out, cutting, excessive sleeping, and the sexual-based issues that I see in my office. These are often based on healing the exile or working with the unconscious. None of this is just going to go away with talk therapy.

Firefighter and Managers Parts are often polarized, not in alignment, and will ultimately cause the person to become stuck and divided. The Manager will criticize the Firefighter's behavior (listed above) making the individual feel bad about themselves.

The Manager if it could talk, would say, "I can't believe you did that. Why did you do that? Now, Jan (or fill in any person's name) looks like a fool, a blubbery idiot, and is never going to have a relationship."

The Firefighter will respond, "I am protecting Jan and not letting in any emotional pain that's locked away and exiled. Leave me the fuck alone; I must distract her now. Don't you get it, **THAT'S MY JOB!** And I am not going to let her down. Leave me alone."

Both protective Parts are trying to help and have positive intentions; they are trying to distract the person in the only way they know how. Frequently these Parts after an IFS session will let go of their protective role as each Part had been protecting the client, but often doing so in a contradictory way.

I will use Dr. Anderson's definition of a Firefighter, a reactive or extreme Part he writes, "A protective Part that typically emerges after a wounded Part is triggered. Firefighters respond in an extreme and sometimes overreactive fashion, typically don't care about the well-being of others, and responses include sui-cide, cutting, drinking, binging, raging, shaming, and dissociating" (p. 7).

Exiles: The Wounded Parts

Protectors work so hard because of Exiles, which are the wounded Parts of us that carry the pain of the original injuries, distress, and emotional or attachment wounds from the past and childhood. They are called "Exiles" because they are banished from the system's conscious awareness by the Protectors. Exile parts are stuck in the time when the physical or emotional injury occurred.

Dr. Anderson writes that this wounded Part, "carries painful thoughts, feelings, and physical sensations because of traumatic or overwhelming expe-riences. The client expends a great deal of energy to keep exiled parts out of conscious awareness. Examples include Parts that feel alone, unloved, shamed, or worthless" (p. 7).

Metaphor for IFS and Parts

To use a metaphor in understanding Parts, I will use an analogy of driving a commercial bus across the country. To drive a commercial bus, the driver is required to have a Commercial Driving License. The bus is the vehicle (the physical body of a human). The people sitting in the seats represent the various Parts, and the Self would be the wise being with the license who is in charge of driving the bus from one state to another. On this particular bus, many of the people (Parts) sitting in the seats believe they have the skills to drive a large and oversized recreational vehicle, or RVs, and even think they are better drivers than the individual who is in charge and driving with the appropriate license.

If there is a major roadblock—one without a police officer detail to direct the bus—the passengers may not feel safe. On this bus, one of the passen-gers, a Manager Part, decides the licensed driver can't handle it and opts to take over. The reason the Manager Part was so determined to do this was because it suffered from an unconscious memory long forgotten of a similar time when a similar experience happened. The Manager's autonomic nerv-ous system enters the flight state, and it must mobilize in some way. It now thinks the driver is unable to handle the situation, and only the Manager can handle the situation with self-assurance, self-confidence, and believes it is completely composed.

When the Manager finds it really can't handle the event, the Firefighter quickly runs to the front of the bus, pushes the Manager aside, and takes over the driving. It believes it is helping by taking control of the incident. Like a real firefighter, hired to run into burning buildings to save those inside, this firefighting Part rushes in to help without consideration of what is happening around it. This causes a total disruption for the rest of the passengers on the bus, the Exiles.

The Exiles become overwhelmed, some scream, others freeze, and still others go into a state of shock. The Firefighter looks in the rearview mirror, sees the Exiles, and notices all their pain. This causes the Firefighter to press the gas, go faster, and ultimately lose all control. This is when the bus hits a tree, causing huge amounts of collateral damage. While this bus was fast-moving, it sideswiped other cars, trucks, and even ran over people who were seriously hurt.

When the investigation occurs, it is established Self is cleared of any wrongdoing because he was not able to drive the bus due to the reactive Protectors who overtook the bus without any notice. The Exiles were found completely comatose; they were shocked back into their original wounded state. Unfortunately, the bus itself loses and is impounded.

This metaphor is a helpful way to look at many of the reactions or behaviors I see in my office. I especially feel compassion for my OCSB clients who struggle with their Firefighters. Frequently, these individuals are men who have partners who don't understand the man's behavior and metaphorically condemn the individual to jail, to live alone, or to live a life without support. You will read in this book some men unwillingly had to divorce their partners, discussed in the story of Billy in Chapter 11.

Integrative Neuro Linguistic Programming (INLP) and Parts

INLP has its foundation in Neuro Linguistic Programming (NLP) which is a psychological approach used by many successful individuals to reach personal goals. Richard Bandler, an information scientist and mathematician, and John Grinder, a linguist, are known for the development of NLP in the early 1970s. NLP is a tool that can be effective in assisting individuals in reaching personal goals.

Much of NLP's footings are based on the work of three talented individuals in the field of psychology. Virginia Satir, a family therapist who practiced in the 1970s, Fritz Perls, who founded Gestalt Therapy (enhanced awareness of sensations in the body, emotions, and behaviors in the present moment), and Milton Erickson, a 20th-century psychiatrist who specialized in hypnosis. I would add a fourth person, Dr. Richard Schwartz, and his work in the 1980s. Of course, all this work hinges on the findings of Carl Jung, who worked from the beginning to the mid-1900s.

In the book, *You Must Learn NLP: 156 Ways of learning Neuro Linguistic Programming Will Improve Your Life,* Dr. Heidi Herron and Laureli Blyth write, "Neuro Linguistic Programming (NLP) is a grouping of concepts, methodology, and skills to help you understand how the language of the mind creates programs you run in your life. The actual definition of NLP will vary from person to person, because you will read in this book, NLP can be so many things" (p. xv in the introduction).

NLP comprehends the value of working with the mind and neurology. This modality brings the concept to the cellular level; it discusses the five senses at a non-verbal level. There is a term coined by Dr. Stephen Porges, "neuroception," which describes the five senses and how they inform the autonomic nervous system (ANS). The ANS just seems to "know" what to do through the various nerve pathways in the body.

Herron and Blyth write about this, "every single thing you've ever seen, said, tasted, touched, smelled, thought, or felt is within your awareness. Automatically, what has come into your awareness connects with your neurology: based on the internal or external stimuli, your brain creates and secretes chemicals, hormones, and neurotransmitters that instantly trigger your unconscious programming and you have a physical, mental, or emotional reaction. Instantly" (pp. xv–xvi).

When I read that, a Part of me was feeling the energy of my own excitement, my ANS was sympathetically aroused and I felt my heart pounding faster, my breath growing deeper, and I became energized. So much of what I'd learned and practiced over the years coalesced when I read Heron and Blyth's work, confirming my deep appreciation of the process. For years, I understood how neuroception influences the ANS, causing the body to go into a stressed state of flight or fight, impacting the individual to feel strained, tensed, and anxious. All of this resulted in an individual's Firefighter parts trying to regulate, by accessing unwanted behavior like OCSB. Or perhaps it shows up, somaticized as vaginismus, discussed in the IFS section of this chapter. Neuroscience was now recognizing parts that are triggered at the unconscious level, by another modality, NLP.

What I appreciate most about Herron and Blyth's definition is the concept of how various modalities or psychological concepts in NLP can and do vary once they become established techniques. For example, I studied INLP, developed by Dr. Matt James, founder of Empowerment Inc., an organization specializing in alternative and integrative approaches to psychology, human understanding, and personal growth. In his model INLP he merges both psychological, and neurological sciences, and integrates Hawaiian spiritual teaching, whereas NLP doesn't include the spiritual component. I have seen this with other modalities, EMDR, the enneagram, and other therapeutic techniques where practitioners place their own lens on the modality to teach their version. I have done this with IFS; I developed the IFS and sandtray model that I named, "IFSsandtray" shown in the work I have done with Jane in chapters twelve and thirteen.

In my foundational INLP training we covered, "Parts Integration," a basic section of the NLP training. IFS would call this a polarization, where two Parts have different agendas and opposite views on what is going to be the most helpful for the system. Often, strong, and conflicting Parts—one a manager, the other is a Firefighter—have positive intentions yet go about it in contradictory ways.

In the NLP framework, the individual is in a state of conflict, each Part is held in the unconscious mind, is to be taken literally, is considered to be a neural network, and—similarly to IFS—the Parts act independently from the whole. The whole in IFS is Self and in Porge's Polyvagal Theory this would be considered the calm and centered state where curiosity occurs when a person is in the ventral vagal state. See chapter six which integrates both IFS and the Polyvagal Theory. While in conflict, the ANS would be in a state of flight or fight state of being, one of mobilization or movement.

In the INLP training manual, the word "Part" is defined, "any state-dependent neural network with enough functional autonomy to run its strategies without control by the rest of the mind." NLP breaks this down to three areas (p. 66). First, the Part becomes activated when an individual is in a triggering situation. This would be the state of preparing to move the body for the ANS. Secondly, there is a neural network that is within the unconscious mind which contributes to the physical behaviors, Default Mode Network's (DMN) negating belief—which we know is wired in the brain, from Dr. Jeffery Rediger and Dr. Daniel Siegel's work listed above. Thirdly, the Part acts independently and may not have the whole system's best intentions, or in IFS, the Parts are not acting with calm, clarity, or any form of connectedness. They are in the Protector mode of a Manager (proactive) or Firefighter (reactive), thus causing polarization.

In the healing process, both IFS and NLP have curative ways to address these issues and I have found both modalities helpful. It is not in the scope of this book to discuss the methodology of how each therapeutic lens restores and integrates the parts, but I find both beneficial tools.

Reference

Anderson, F. G., *Transcending trauma: Healing complex PTSD with internal family systems therapy*. PESI Publishing, Eau Claire, WI, 2021 (pp. 7–8).

Adaptive Defenses to Use on the Journey   **6**

Using Internal Family Systems Through the Polyvagal Theory Lens

Entering an in-depth therapeutic process is very much an individual journey. Many may seek answers from others, but so often superfluous comments, insights, and annotations prove unhelpful; it was the other person's exploration for the answers, not their own. To really seek the truth, they must go inside themselves and ask the hard questions. These self-inquiries are a challenging, overwhelming undertaking. This inner exploration requires a serious commitment to oneself, presenting unique challenges. True, life-enhancing healing must happen from the inside out. Completing an in-depth psychotherapy treatment process demands continuous inner focus, comprehensive awareness of one's emotions, and a physical state of being. This soul-finding endeavor is, to me, the hero's journey.

The hero's journey begins when someone chooses to leave the familiar behind, accepting the need to go into the unknown to heal something inside. Frequently, this requires a mentor, someone to help navigate the unfamiliar. This trusted individual can help the hero deal with difficulties and transform the expedition. An initial spark of self-awareness, courage, and the desire to change is required to embark on this process of transformation, to achieve wholeness; it is not Minotaurs or dragons that need slaying, but something else, buried deep within. For these intrepid explorers, the hero's journey begins in an office (nowadays, often not in person, but via Zoom) with a therapist. It is in

DOI: 10.4324/9781003388302-7

this setting that the pioneers learn to navigate difficult situations or events, unraveling trauma that may have originated in early childhood, and healing from core negative beliefs.

There has to be a moment of insight for the hero, our clients, to know when unhelpful behavioral patterns arise. These clients, when confounded by anxiety and distress seek the relief only therapists (mentors) can provide. The first sparks of self-awareness are often ignited early in the journey by the individual showing enough curiosity to want to notice, identify, and explore the very emotions and behaviors causing them distress.

The dragons lurk within. By utilizing the concepts of Internal Family Systems (IFS) through the lens of the Polyvagal Theory (PVT) one can clearly see that these difficult emotions and behaviors are adaptive defenses. It is important to recognize how the IFS model accepts that all emotions (called Parts) have positive intentions to help the person. Every IFS clinician knows that all individuals have what is known as Self in the IFS model. Self is not a Part but a state of being where a person is calm, curious, compassionate, and sees the world with clarity, confidence, and creativity—they are connected to themselves and others. In addition, this state of being includes patience, perspective, persistence, playfulness, and perseverance. In the PVT those qualities also exist as a state of being known as Ventral vagal.

The PVT informs us the autonomic nervous system (ANS) reacts to any and all situations instantaneously and in milliseconds without any conscious thought as it reacts to perceived and actual threats. This often causes Parts to become activated and engage to protect the system in ways that, from the outside looking in, don't seem very helpful. IFS clarifies how Parts also act in response to situations to protect the system from both physical and emotional pain. In some pronounced cases, the individual may experience various extreme reactions resulting in behaviors such as Out of Control Sexual Behavior (OCSB), also referred to as problematic sexual behavior. In some cases, the individual may react with suicidal ideation, cutting, numbing with street drugs, or misusing prescription medication, substance abuse, gambling, and anger and rage. It is the ANS that stimulates the Parts to engage, resulting in behaviors to *assist* the body in trying to mobilize back to a state of Ventral vagal in the PVT and Self in IFS.

Unfortunately, these behaviors don't help and often hurt the individual. People enter our offices wounded, often possessing beliefs about themselves such as, "I can't be trusted," "I don't deserve love," "I am not good enough," and others like "it's not okay to feel or show my emotions." These core negative beliefs are held by Parts that exist within each of the PVT states.

In the PVT there is a mobilizing state called Sympathetic. It is there where reactive protector Parts (called Firefighters in the IFS model) step in to take control. Firefighters are willing to do anything to avoid feeling any emotional pain; they are reactive, impulsive, often controlling, rebellious, self-harming, and do not appear helpful at all.

There is another protective type of Part that appears to be proactive but mobilizes in a completely different way than the Firefighter. These protective Parts are called Managers and also reside in the mobilizing state of Sympathetic. Managers, unlike Firefighters, won't be reactive, but rather go into a proactive mode of being productive, problem solving, helpful, preparing for difficult situations in advance, and often taking on responsibilities. Their beliefs are "I get things done," "I take care of others," "I will complete things perfectly," and they usually follow societal norms. This, for example, can look like a perfectionist, which can be overwhelming. That is when the Firefighters engage to stop the overwhelming feelings. Once in this reactive state, the individual will appear to go into a cycle where they engage in behaviors that don't regulate them, such as those mentioned above. Too many people, including therapists, label this as "addiction;" I call it a dysregulated ANS.

When the ANS is dysregulated, the defensive behaviors of the Firefighter can't bring the individual back into Self or ventral vagal state, which was its original positive intent. Instead, what happens is the system often goes into a collapsed or dissociative state. This is one of two immobilized states. This disintegrated state is known as the dorsal vagal in the PVT. The other immobilized state is where a person is regulated, sleeps peacefully, allowing a non-triggered state of rest and restore.

The dorsal vagal state is where the individual is completely shut down. It's not an exact match to the IFS model of the Part known as an Exile which holds emotional pain from the original traumatizing or upsetting event. These Parts hold the qualities of feeling invisible, sadness, broken-heartedness, guilt, shame, disconnected, overwhelmed, and despondent. They hold the beliefs of "I am weak, worthless, permanently damaged, and deeply depressed."

Knowing IFS through the PVT lens broadens our comprehension of how human beings seem to transform their personality within a very short time frame, from easygoing and secure one moment to angry or insecure a split second later. This, then, leads to the feeling that they are helpless or powerless in a situation.

When we look at our clients as having Parts and an ANS together, one realizes they are comprised of two protective systems: one psychological (IFS) and the other physiological (PVT). Since the ANS is physiological, it can't hold beliefs about itself, whereas Parts can, as if they are like little human beings with varying emotions ultimately influencing a person's beliefs about themselves.

With this understanding, I designed one chart and four graphics, inserted below, which display how Parts in the IFS modality align closely to the states in the PVT. The chart is an overall image, and the four graphics are illustrations shown with miniatures (Table 6.1).

These visual aids illustrate how human beings have defense systems that work in tandem. In addition, they illustrate how the ANS has enormous effects on a human being's emotions and behaviors. It appears that Parts hold many core beliefs; these convictions depend on what state they exist in, in the ANS. This information can support therapists and their clients alike. The first one, Figure 6.1, represents the Self in IFS and Ventral Vagal in the PVT.

Table 6.1 Polyvagal and IFS Chart

Polyvagal Theory (PVT)	Internal Family Systems (IFS)
Ventral Vagal	Self (Inner peace)
• Tranquil • Reflective • Enthusiastic • Lively • Proficient	• Balanced • Connected • Hopeful • Playful • Flexible
Sympathetic (Proactive mobilization)	Managers (Beliefs)
• Accountable • Cooperative • Supportive • Compliant • Tolerant • Persistent	• I get things done • I have control • I take care of others • I will complete things perfectly • I am prepared
Sympathetic (Reactive mobilization)	Firefighters (Beliefs)
• Combative • Thoughtless • Impetuous • Reckless • Impulsive	• I cannot be trusted • I am out of control • I am not good enough • It's not safe to show my emotions
Dorsal Vagal (Immobilization)	Exiles (Beliefs)
• Shutdown • Disengaged • Detached • Speechless • Disoriented • Bewildered	• I am worthless • I am permanently damaged • I am broken • I am powerless • I am shameful • I am helpless

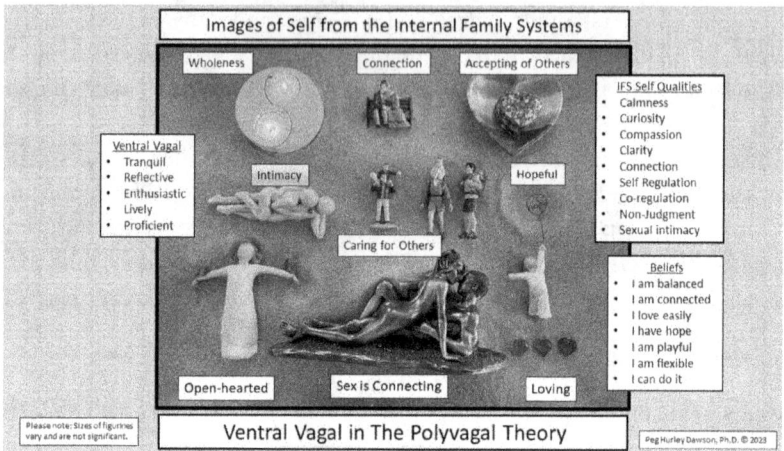

Figure 6.1 Self and Ventral Vagal

Photo by the author

The image represents Self in IFS, or Ventral Vagal in PVT, a state of *being* rather than *doing*. Self and ventral vagal are feelings of safety, a relaxed way of being in the body and the world. This is when human beings are aligned with themselves, others, and even beyond. This is an inner knowing, an embodied sense where the "C" qualities in IFS exist: calm, curious, clarity, courage, compassion, connectedness, confidence, and curiosity. It also represents the five "p's" in IFS: patience, presence, persistence, perspective, and playfulness. This is where nothing must be done, fixed, changed, and one is at peace with themselves and nature.

When an individual's ANS senses or perceives a situation as dangerous it will move instantaneously out of the ventral vagal a centered state, into a mobilizing state of the ANS, called the Sympathetic nervous system—which prepares the body's flight or fight response when there is a perceived threat. When an individual doesn't feel safe, the sympathetic system automatically prepares the body to mobilize, engaging the two types of Protectors in the IFS model.

The next two images are of the mobilizing state of sympathetic arousal where mobilization and the flight/fight response occur. Two images are required to express this state because there is a significant difference from how human beings react to various situations. One is proactive and the other reactive. In PVT there is a mobilizing response. In IFS there are two types of mobilized Parts, known as Managers, who appear to be proactive in how they deal with issues. The others are Firefighters who are reactive in how they deal with situations (Figure 6.2).

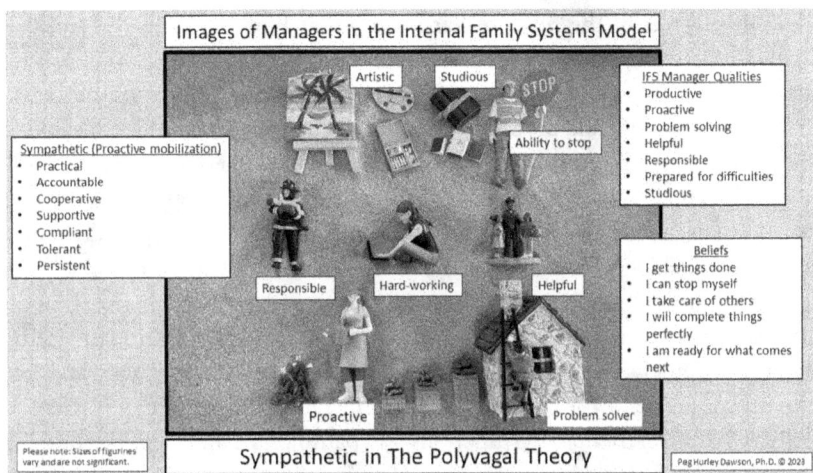

Figure 6.2 Managers and Sympathetic

Photo by the author

This image is of the protective Parts known as Managers in IFS, and the state of sympathetic in the PVT. Here the individual may feel like they are getting things done efficiently, and often displaying the qualities of being productive, exhibiting the ability to problem solve, be helpful, and responsible. They are being proactive and managing situations effectively (Figure 6.3).

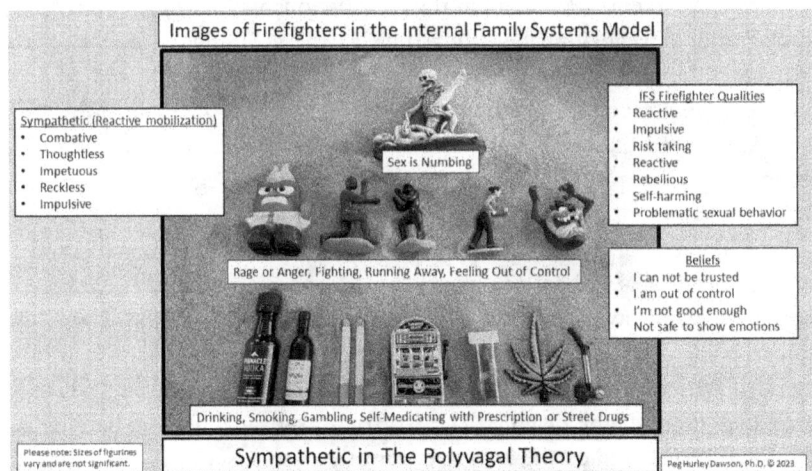

Figure 6.3 Firefighters and Sympathetic

Photo by the author

This image is of the reactive Parts known as Firefighters in IFS and the sympathetic state in the PVT. These reactive Parts often express behaviors such as hyper-vigilance, bullying, rebelling, dominating, anxiety, and others. In addition, I would add problematic Sexual Behavior. In my office, a sympathetic behavior often displayed is OCSB. OCSB is defined as when the individual feels out of control. OCSB is a Firefighter; unfortunately, sometimes it doesn't make any sense how this behavior might be helpful—especially when it leads to a behavior that a person hates or one that hurts their partner.

The individual who is reactive may feel they must react to a situation or numb themselves with alcohol, gambling, drugs, and sex. Often these methods are extremely unhelpful in solving any situation. These protective Parts often result in chaos for the individual. Some clinicians, who may not know IFS or PVT, label them as dysfunctions and pathologize the client rather than understanding this is the Part's reactivity in protecting an original wound called an Exile in IFS.

Reactivity can be understood differently when we observe it in the context of sympathetic overwhelm in response to perceived or real danger. This get-up-and-go momentum may not be recognized consciously yet it drives a compelling need for physical action. I would also like to add that the individual who uses any maladaptive coping mechanisms—OCSB or problematic sexual behavior, or any of the reactive Protectors—is most likely a repercussive result from an experience of trauma or attachment wound from early childhood. In all cases, the ANS is perceiving danger in that moment.

These past events are stored in the unconscious which triggers the ANS, resulting in dysregulating behavior such as these Firefighters or reactive Protective Parts. As a reminder, all Parts have positive intents and, in this case, reactive protectors are trying desperately to protect the Exile or the Part that experienced the original wound from a trauma (such as an attachment wound, mental or physical abuse, or neglect). Shown in Figure 6.4 Exiles and Dorsal Vagal

This image is of the wounded Parts known as Exiles in IFS and is in the state of dorsal vagal in the PVT. These "hurt Parts" often are unable to express themselves as behaviors because they are in a collapsed state. In this state in human beings, the prefrontal cortex is offline, as well as any desire to mobilize. It is where an individual feels disconnected, completely overwhelmed, and experiences shame or guilt. The words, dorsal vagal may be familiar to many who have studied the PVT, yet for others, this is a foreign concept. I once used those words in a paper to describe a client's state, sent the paper to an editor, and he wrote back, "what does this mean your client was on his back?" I laughed out loud because that is what dorsal literally means and

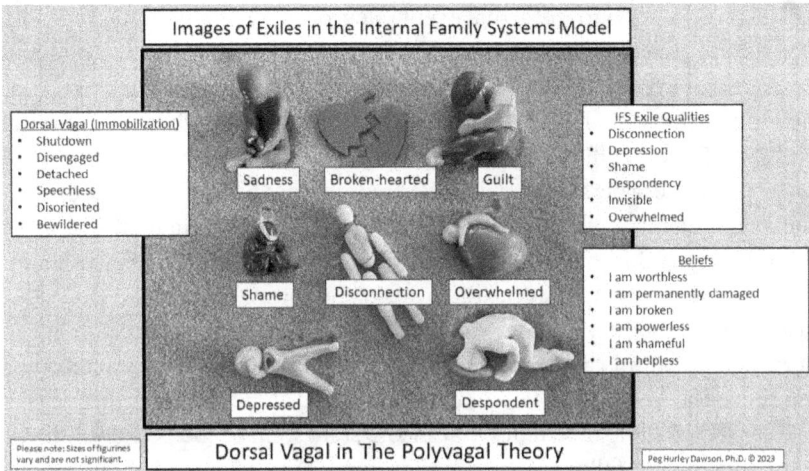

Figure 6.4 Exiles and Dorsal Vagal

Photo by the author

I had not even thought of this interpretation. This also illustrates the need to understand the concept, using clinical terms sparingly, to avoid confusion with your clients.

Dorsal vagal is a state of the ANS, described by Deb Dana in her book, *The Polyvagal Theory: Engaging in the Rhythm of Regulation* (2018). In it, she writes, "Our primitive dorsal vagal circuit, 500 million years old, protects through immobilization, shutting down the body systems to conserve energy, similar to the way that animals feign death in response to life-threat ('playing possum')" (p. 19).

Dorsal vagal is part of the Parasympathetic Nervous System, sometimes written in scientific literature as PNS. Deb Dana (2018) describes this succinctly, "The origin of the dorsal vagal pathway of the parasympathetic branch and its immobilization responses lies with our ancient vertebrate ancestors and is the oldest pathway" (p. 9). The PNS is one of the two branches of the ANS. One branch of the PNS (ventral vagal) engages whenever human beings feel and perceive safety, meaning is able to rest comfortably and with ease, digest food, feel calm, and their heart rate lowers; the other branch (dorsal vagal) engages in times of extreme danger.

To give a more detailed example of how an individual moves quickly into any of the states an analogy may be in order. A perceived threat occurs when a person has had a life experience where the danger was real, and the body linked a sound, sight, smell, touch, or taste, one or more of the five senses called neuroception to the actual event. Neuroception is a word Dr. Stephen Porges, the creator of PVT coined as there wasn't any other word that could describe this event. Neuroception happens within milliseconds and occurs at the unconscious level. The memory is held within the individual's physical body (PVT), and in IFS, the Part's body.

For example, a person in an abusive environment hears the sounds of footsteps on a staircase which means that their abuser is coming up the stairs to harm them. In this example, the person was abused, and the ANS will connect the auditory system, recalling this as dangerous whenever the individual hears a similar sound. Another example is when a veteran returns after active duty. A loud boom can trigger the ANS to respond as if it is an explosion or gunshot. The body/ANS remembers and stores all information through its five senses. In some modalities that incorporate somatic interventions, these sensations can be followed, accessing unconscious, yet powerful, memories just by using body memory.

Early childhood experiences and stressors affect both the body and the Parts. These early life experiences, held as burdens, follow the individual into adulthood, Dr. Frank Anderson (2021) writes, "The wounded parts are the young, sensitive, and vulnerable aspects of our personalities. They were forced to carry the hurt, pain, sense of betrayal, sadness, loneliness, shame, neglect, and lack of love. It is related to the painful and difficult moments in our lives" (p. 18).

In the article, "Timing of Early-Life Stress and the Development of Brain-Related Capacities" the authors write, "Early-life stress (ELS) poses risks for developmental and mental health problems throughout the lifespan" (Vol. 13, Article 183). These mental health issues stem from exiled Parts of the system where it responds physically and emotionally by shutting down completely, or by going into a collapsed or "submit state" shown in Figure 6.4.

References

Anderson, F., *Transcending trauma: Healing complex PTSD with internal family systems therapy*. PESI Publishing, Eau Claire, WI, 2021 (p. 18).

Dana, D., *The polyvagal theory in therapy: Engaging the rhythm of regulation*. W. W. Norton & Company, Inc, New York, NY, 2018 (pp. 9, 18–19).

What Goes in the Backpack? The Four Bs

7

Beliefs, Body, Brain, and Behavior

When new clients call me to see if they can make an appointment, they often tell me they have seen other therapists and want to try someone or something different. Sometimes they let me know their diagnosis, whether the therapist was helpful or not, and without exception, they tell me they want to change in some way. They want to undergo a transformative experience because they haven't been able to realize lasting change.

At some level most of these individuals have experienced upsetting events or traumatic incidents in childhood. Often, they don't know this, and even tell me, "Oh, I didn't have trauma, I had some bad stuff happen but, it wasn't as bad as what other people I know had to go through." When I hear their stories, I know what happened to them was indeed traumatic. These adverse occurrences have consequences resulting in lasting impacts on their physical, emotional, and sexual health, and adverse effects on their relationships.

I am a trauma-informed sex therapist; I often see the negative impact of early childhood trauma displayed in adult sexual behavior, including early or delayed ejaculation, vaginismus, problematic sexual behavior, OCSB, and other sexual issues, showing up in their lives with core negative beliefs. What are core negative beliefs? Think of them as words, when strung together, which may ring true for many clients. Some of them are: "I am not good enough," "I am weak," or even "It's not okay for me to trust myself or anyone else." These

DOI: 10.4324/9781003388302-8

beliefs have grown out of doubt, worry, and feelings of being flawed in some way. I lived with the first one, "I am not good enough," for a long time. No matter what the negative core belief is, it can be healed and reframed. How can I be so sure of that? I healed from mine; I see many individuals heal and reframe theirs, and I see it happen all the time in my practice.

I am also a therapist who works with couples. I have witnessed individuals in their relationship experience core negative beliefs in their adult partnerships. I am always fascinated by how so many people choose someone who is ultimately going to be what Richard Schwartz, the founder of Internal Family Systems, calls, "Tor-Mentors."

In Schwartz's (2008) book, *You Are the One You've Been Waiting For*, he wrote,

> … our partner can be an invaluable tor-mentor—that is, a person who mentors us by tormenting us. It is very difficult to find all our basement children when we're not in an intimate relationship because often we only become aware of them when they are triggered by an intimate partner. Inevitably, our partner will act like an early caretaker who hurts us, and we will have an extreme reaction—and attachment re-injury. If we follow the trail of emotion to its inner source, we will find yet another exile in need of our love.

Frequently we are attracted to partners we believe will accept us as we are, take us away from the heartache of feeling profoundly alone, and they could never emotionally open our deepest wounds. Alas, we also have the potential to choose a person who will hurt us most deeply, often leaving us emotionally depleted from the very injuries which happened in our family of origin. This distress frequently involves trust. In my practice, where I specialize in treating problematic sexual behavior, I see the person some might identify as the "betrayer." I say betrayer not because I think they are a betrayer, but rather because that is often how they, themselves, refer to what they did to their partner or their significant other.

I prefer to think of them as victims of early childhood trauma, desperately trying to find release for their own stressed-out systems. The partner who feels betrayed often doesn't realize they have chosen a "Tor-Mentor" who will ultimately replicate something they have experienced before, by some individual earlier in their life. The ironic thing is when they first meet their significant other, they feel remarkably comfortable, almost like they have known that person for years. This, in many ways, is true. They had most likely, in their own childhood, known someone whose mannerisms are the same as their original caretaker. I have seen this situation a few times, enough to realize it's more typical than not. This ultimately becomes a trust issue.

When any person in a relationship has experienced a challenging family of origin, trust is often impacted, even at a very young age. Unfortunately, this becomes a theme for some individuals in how they behave in relationships with others. When a person is raised in an environment where their trust was broken by a caretaker who couldn't be present, an attachment wound occurs. The emotional dysregulation dance of reenacting early childhood wounds begins.

Let me put this into context with an example of a typical situation I see in my practice. An individual may ask for therapy to heal from problematic sexual behavior. They are often considered betrayers because of their activity of going to massage parlors, viewing sexual imagery, or behaving in some other way to which their partner never consented. The underlying root of this behavior, however, is early childhood attachment wounds, caused by caretakers who may have truly loved them, but due to their own dysregulation, proved unavailable to attune to the child. These young children often do develop core negative beliefs at very young ages.

These negative beliefs are what Dr. Jeffery Rediger referred to in his book, *Cured: The Life-Changing Science of Spontaneous Healing,* as a default mode network (DMN) he writes,

> A more scientific term for it is your default mode network (DMN). The DMN is basically a collection of loosely connected regions of the brain, both older structures deep in the brain and newer ones in the cerebral cortex, which are activated, or light up when you engage in certain categories of thinking.
>
> (Rediger, 2020)

I found default mode network (DMN) frequently holds as core negative beliefs that often happened before the age of five, and I have referred to them as Pro-Symptom Beliefs years before reading Dr. Rediger's book. I use these Pro-Symptom Beliefs to help clients heal from their upsetting events in early childhood and even trauma somatically frozen in time in their bodies (see chapters 8 and 16).

I typically work with two major non-pathologizing frameworks in my practice: the Polyvagal Theory and the Neurosequential Model of Therapeutics. In earlier chapters, I've covered the Polyvagal Theory (PVT). PVT informs us how all human beings have an automatic nervous system that responds to stress and trauma. I also feel it is essential to understand the Neurosequential Model of Therapeutics (NMT), designed by Dr. Bruce Perry, MD, Ph.D., a neuroscientist, researcher, and child psychiatrist.

NMT provides a significant and influential lens for comprehending how early childhood experiences affect human brain development. Research has shown NMT can provide significant insight into treating all individuals. In the 2009 issue of the *Journal of Loss and Trauma*, Dr. Perry writes,

> Because the brain is most plastic (receptive to environmental input) in early childhood, the child is most vulnerable to variance of experience during this time. Again, the clinical, practice, and policy implications are profound.

NMT, similarly to PVT, is not a therapeutic technique or intervention, it is a developmentally sensitive, evidenced-based, and neurobiologically informed approach for understanding the human development of the brain when it is exposed to traumatic or even upsetting events early in life. Remember, some of these upsetting events may not be upsetting to the parent or caregiver, at the time, but to the young child, they establish the long-lasting negative core beliefs that will follow them into adulthood.

A thorough working knowledge of NMT is beneficial for all clinicians, parents, teachers, and anyone interested in understanding brain development. Dr. Perry and Oprah Winfrey (2021) wrote the book on NMT, *What Happened to You? Conversations on Trauma, Resilience, and Healing,* and never once mentioned the words Neurosequential Model of Therapeutics. With its straightforward, non-clinical vocabulary and simple approach, the book made it easy for all people to understand a complex concept. This is one of the books I recommend to clients and students alike, many of whom mentioned how it helped them understand the importance of early childhood experiences which may underly the issues for which they are seeking therapy.

NMT is a model of how the brain develops both anatomically as well as developmentally from the brainstem to the midbrain area, followed by the limbic region, and finally at the apex, the cortex. The brainstem is responsible for the basic necessities of existence including control of blood pressure, heart rate, respiration, and body temperature. This is the first area of the brain to grow in human development. At the brainstem level, the autonomic nervous system is the principal regulator of the five senses. This is called *neuroception* from Dr. Porges' work in the Polyvagal Theory. Neuroception is another word for the five senses present at birth and that allows the infant to "know" when they are safe or not.

In infancy, the individual only has the body to inform the caretaker what is happening. The caretaker's *responses* to the child's actions are critical. How the caretaker responds will determine how the child forms their identity and the core beliefs, mentioned above. If the caretaker is consistently attuned to the child, they will feel valued. If the caretaker isn't attuned, for whatever reason, the child will develop negative beliefs about themselves. Gabor Mate in his 2022 book, *The Myth of Normal: Trauma, Illness & Healing in a Toxic Culture* writes,

> Especially in infancy, but throughout childhood, the young human uses the emotional and nervous systems of the caring adults to regulate their own internal states. The interpersonal-biological math is elementary: the more stressed the adult, the more stressed the child.
>
> (Mate & Mate, 2022, p. 169)

In the same text Dr. Mate addresses how early childhood trauma often results in adults developing shame-based core beliefs he writes,

> People bearing trauma's scars almost uniformly develop a shame-based view of themselves at the core, a negative self-perception most of them are all too conscious of. Among the most poisonous consequence of shame is the loss of compassion for oneself. The more severe the trauma, the more total that loss.
>
> (Mate & Mate, 2022, p. 30)

Self-compassion is a foundational element in healing for adults, especially those who have experienced early childhood upsetting events, trauma, and mis-attunement in childhood.

If an individual is raised in an unpredictable and chaotic environment, their autonomic nervous system (ANS) reacts as if the world is dangerous and has always been. When the ANS senses danger, it will react by sending adrenaline, a hormone secreted into the body by the adrenal glands. This happens to both children and adults, and when an individual feels stressed, their blood pressure increases, heart rate elevates, triggering the flight or fight response.

Often, the flight or fight response occurs when a human is unable to self soothe and their autonomic nervous system reacts in a stimulated, energized, and mobilizing state, also known as sympathetic arousal. Many times, this is due to early childhood upsetting events, traumas, mis-attunement, by original caretakers, children often become dysregulated adults who are unable to self-soothe. When a human being is unable to self soothe, their autonomic nervous systems are often in the aroused or energized state known as sympathetic often referred to as the flight and fight state. This may cause issues for the adult sexually, resulting in problematic sexual behavior or other mental health issues. It can even appear as attention-deficit disorder (ADD).

To emphasize how parents can have an impact in Attention Deficit Disorder in their children, Gabor Mate writes in *Scattered: How Attention Deficit Disorder Originates and What You Can Do About It,*

> Parents may need to change their lifestyles, sacrificing whatever activities can be eliminated if these diminish their availability to their ADD child. This could mean saying no and disappointing friends or colleagues, and it might mean giving up projects and involvements close to one's heart. There is a lot to be gained, however, for their child has already incurred a deficit of attention.
>
> (Mate, 2000)

Note how Dr. Mate speaks in terms of deficit of attention, not attention deficit disorder.

The second level is the midbrain, where sleep, appetite/satiety, and arousal are controlled. The midbrain is the limbic area, which manages motor regulation, emotional reactivity, and sexual behaviors.

At the apex is the largest section: the cortical area. This is where abstract thought and concrete thought are held. This is the area that makes human beings different from other mammals. This is the last section of the brain to develop. To quote the title of the book, it is all about *what happened to you* that determines the outcome of how the cortex will be formed and ultimately how an individual learns their own core beliefs. See Figure 7.1.

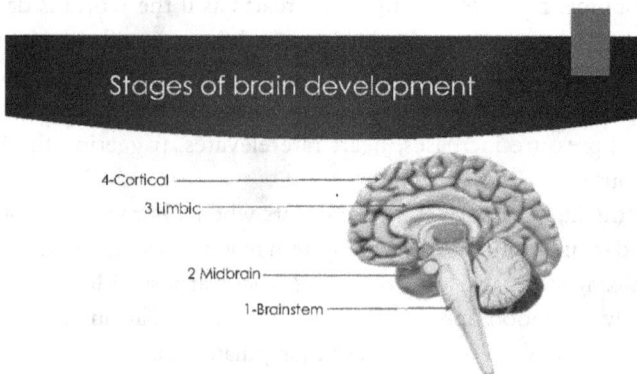

Figure 7.1 Stages of Brain Development

Image Created by the author

Dr. Perry's on-line webinars, the NMT perspective, and his informative YouTube videos provide significant background on the many ways early childhood trauma can affect every relationship in adulthood. Ironically it is in a relationship with another where our childhood traumas re-emerge and cause us to experience heartache. It is in the heartache many of us seek to understand why our partner could make us feel so bad. This often brings us into therapy. Therapy is where we can access the unconscious right brain to heal negative core beliefs which often stem from early childhood mis-attunement, upsetting experiences, or traumatic events. When those wounds heal, couples no longer need to recreate the earliest childhood wounds in their adult relationships. In Chapter 9 I will cover how the NMT model has been applied to Kalffian Sandplay.

References

Mate, G., Scattered: How attention deficit disorder originates and what you can do about it. First plume printing, August 2000. Penguin Group, New York, NY, 2000 (p. 175).

Mate, G., & Mate, D., *The myth of normal: Trauma, illness & healing in a toxic culture*. Penguin Random House LLC, New York, NY, 2022 (p. 30).

Mate, G., & Mate, D., *The myth of normal: Trauma, illness & healing in a toxic culture*. Penguin Random House LLC, New York, NY, 2022 (p. 169).

Perry, B. D., & Winfrey, O., *What happened to you? Conversations on trauma, resilience, and healing*. Flatiron Books, New York, 2021.

Rediger, J., *Cured: The life-changing science of spontaneous healing*. Flatiron Books, New York, NY, 2020 (p. 269).

Schwartz, R., *You are the one you've been waiting for*. Trailheads Publications, Boulder CO, 2008 (p. 95).

Accessing the   **8**
Unconscious Mind
Using Metaphor, Sandplay, and IFSsandtray

A client came to me because she was having difficulty with sexual intimacy due to chronic neck pain, which prevented her from pleasurable experiences. During an IFSsandtray session, she found a Part of herself that thought her partner was basically a pain in the neck. In this instance, what the body is telling us is hardly subtle. But sometimes the signals the body is sending us aren't so easily interpreted. The body communicates with us regularly, but we don't always understand what it's telling us and why we are feeling this way. Many times, these symptoms are metaphors or messages from the unconscious. I've observed the physical body manifesting problems stemming from unconscious beliefs so often that now, whether I am working in sand or not, I think in metaphors.

This approach, as well as accessing the unconscious in sand work to heal the body and mind, has revolutionized my therapeutic approach and therapy practice. I now trust my clients' unconscious to heal them from the very issues for which they contact me. Most have been in therapy before and are looking for something uniquely different than talking things out. Often, what they hear in the first session with me are words they have never heard from any therapist before. I say, "When we are talking, we're leaning on the left hemisphere of the brain which solves mathematical and scientific problems beautifully. To achieve the kind of healing you are looking for, we need to access the right hemisphere as well—the world of images, metaphors, body sensations of both mental and physically held experiences—sandtray and sandplay can help you with that."

DOI: 10.4324/9781003388302-9

It's not that I don't talk to my clients about important events in their lives or their reactions to those situations. I do. But, I don't want to waste a moment of their time by repeating something I have come to learn isn't helpful. I want to push beyond left-hemisphere thinking and the cycle of talk therapy. As many know, this part of the brain is logical, linguistic, and linear. Once we move beyond talk and into the metaphorical realm, by accessing the right hemisphere, we can find new ways to heal upsetting or traumatic events. I depend on the right hemisphere and somatic bodily sensations to heal people from the inside out—finding a deeper dimension to access the unconscious that may not be available through verbal language alone. I offer a service to my clients that invites them into a new world, where their inner lives can emerge through sandtray, Kalffian sandplay, and metaphor. And I believe I'm part of a growing movement of therapists branching out, embracing new therapeutic methods to access the unconscious through artistic techniques.

Early on, I shared with my clients my trust in a process that will help them heal in a way that they have never tried before. I invite them to trust in themselves and their own unconscious. Given the proper conditions, the brain has the unique ability to solve problems creatively.

Another way we access the unconscious and the right hemisphere is through our dreams. Symbols appear to us in dreams, this of course is not new. Freud talked about the nature of dreams in the 2019 edition of the book titled, *On Dreams*. He wrote:

> Dream symbolism leads us far beyond the dream; it does not belong only to dreams, but is likewise dominant in legend, myth, and saga in wit and folklore. It compels us to pursue the inner meaning of the dream .... But we must acknowledge that symbolism is not a result of the dream work, but is a peculiarity probably of our unconscious thinking ....
>
> (p. 43)

I have come to pay attention to my dreams and those of my clients because that is often where the metaphors and symbolism occur to us in action. This understanding was amplified in the book, *Man and His Symbols,* which was edited by M. I. von Franz after the death of Carl Jung: "Jung discovered that dreams can also give civilized man the guidance he needs in finding his way through the problems of both his inner and his outer life. Indeed, many of our dreams are concerned with details of our outer life and our surroundings" (1964, p. 220).

Another client who came to me originally for out of control sexual behavior worked mostly in the modality of sandplay, and healed from his OCSB in about a year. One day a few years later, he called me and asked me if we could meet again for a few more sessions because he was losing his erections when he was making love with his wife.

When he came in, I suggested using the modality of Kalffan sandplay with him and he readily agreed. Something unique happened in that sandplay session when he selected eight miniatures: a wooden chest, a cage, a brontosaurus, a tealight candle—which he lit—a stone curved staircase, a wavy wire round structure that was open on the top, and two tents. He placed one tent in the upper right corner of the tray and the other one diagonally opposite in the lower left-hand corner.

After he placed all the miniatures into the tray, he said to me, "Peg, I have no idea why I picked any of these miniatures. Or why I felt it was important to pick up *two tents*." His voice accentuated the words, "two tents" which somehow seemed important to notice at the time. I contemplated what possible metaphor the unconscious was trying to symbolically show him. He unconsciously selected the emphasis on the words, *two tents*. I reflected on this and how the two hemispheres work collaboratively. The right brought into consciousness the symbols of the two tents. The left brain used language to emphasize them.

It wasn't until after he left when I was taking photographs to document his work, that it came to me. I experienced a brainwave of what I saw in his sandplay that I wanted to share with him. Flabbergasted, I called him immediately. He answered the phone right away, by now only minutes from the office.

"Are you feeling stressed out lately when you and Helen are being sexually intimate?"

He immediately replied, "Yes, I am, and I really don't know why."

I ventured further, choosing my words carefully. "Are you finding yourself too tense and not relaxed when you are with her lately?

"Yes, I have been tense lately now that I think of it. Why do you ask?"

"I asked you this because you literally selected *two tents* and couldn't comprehend why. I think the importance of picking the two tents might be your psyche's way of showing your conscious mind you need to relax a little bit more because you are *too tense*." He got it immediately and we both laughed.

Word play in metaphor combined with active listening from an attuned and present therapist can change how any clinician may work therapeutically with their clients. What is captured in the example above is not just the word play, but in fact was that I was actively listening. This is why talk is important in conjunction with metaphor, and an active listener is critical in the therapeutic environment. The answer is always in the room, it's just not the clinician who has it. The client can heal many of their physical, sexual, and mental health issues, they simply don't know it yet.

On May 26, 2021, The Trauma Research Foundation in Brookline, Massachusetts ran the 32nd Annual Boston International Trauma Conference where Dr. Lorraine Freedle, then president of Sandplay Therapists of America (STA) presented. Dr. van der Kolk is a well-known researcher in the treatment of trauma and the founder and medical director of the Trauma Research Foundation. He is also the highly respected author of a *New York Times* number one best-selling book, *The Body Keeps the Score: Brain, Mind, and Body in the Healing of Trauma*. That book has been read by many professional trauma researchers, therapists, psychiatrists, and others who are interested in gaining a more complete understanding of how to treat people who suffer from complex trauma. *The Body Keeps the Score* doesn't mention any form of working with sand, a method of healing trauma. Sandplay research was emerging at that time and not readily available for inclusion in his book. Although sandtray research remains in its infancy, sandplay research has rapidly developed in recent years (Wiersma et al. 2022).

Dr. van der Kolk's endorsement of sandplay and sandtray has since been demonstrated by his keynote addresses at various conferences. Additionally, international sandplay teacher Dr. Lorraine Freedle is on the faculty in his traumatic studies certification program. On November 7, 2021, I attended a sandtray conference where he was the keynote presenter and he enthusiastically supported the clinicians using sand in the treatment of trauma.

The neuroscience of sandplay is discussed in the *Journal of Sandplay Therapy* in an article written in 2019 by Dr. Lorraine Freedle. Freedle's research incorporated the work of Dr. Bruce Perry's Neurosequential Model of Therapeutics, Antonio Damasio's theory of consciousness of "Self-Processes," and examples of sandplay therapy activities and themes, these are shown in Table 8.1.

In the same article, Dr. Freedle's Sandplay's Sensory Feedback Loop is also reviewed, documenting the importance of how sandplay therapy is regulating and transformational, shown in Chart 8.1 (used with the author's permission). To further illustrate her examples, I have also included images of two of my client's sand trays—where both regulated themselves purely by moving the sand with their hands, and, in one case, with their feet.

Table 8.1 displays the brain systems and related functions starting at the brainstem, diencephalon, limbic system, and finally, the neocortex shown in the same chapter. The next column in the graphic is labeled, "Clinical Symptoms" illustrating the core symptoms of trauma in the brainstem and

Table 8.1 Neurosequential Model of Therapeutics and Sandplay Therapy Chart

Neurosequential Model of Therapeutics			Antonio Damasio's Theory of Consciousness "Self-Processes"	Examples of Sandplay Therapy Activates/Themes
Brain Region	Clinical symptoms	Functional Domain		
Brain & Diencephalon	Trauma Core Symptoms (brainstem) Depressive and Affect Symptoms (diencephalon)	"Regulate" Sensory Integration & Self-Regulation	"protoself" (unconscious) primordial feelings (felt body states) "material me"	Sensory play Massaging the sand, touching, smoothing Rhythmic, bilateral movements Placing stones or mosaics one-by-one Molding, watering, sifting, constructing Pounding, dumping, flooding, destroying Posttraumatic play, "implicit surges" Use of creepy crawlers, snakes, monsters (devouring or protective aspects
Limbic System	Relational Difficulties Alcohol, Substance Abuse	"Relate" Relational Functioning	"core self" (stable, conscious) internal states "mapped" with perception of objects (thalamocortical links) subjectivity begins emotions, salience	creative play symbolic expression therapeutic relationship, countertransference emotions, desires attachment themes (e.g., nurturing, feeding, abandonment, neglect) use of animals (instincts, emotions, companions)

(Continued)

Table 8.1 Continued

Neurosequential Model of Therapeutics			Antonio Damasio's Theory of Consciousness "Self-Processes"	Examples of Sandplay Therapy Activates/Themes
Brain Region	**Clinical symptoms**	**Functional Domain**		
Neocortex	• Guilt and Shame	*"Reason"* Cognitive Problem Solving	"autobiographical self" elaborately coordinates "pulses" from core self past-present-future extended consciousness "sociocultural and spiritual me"	storytelling, language journey trays reflection, self-awareness, discovery meaning making, insight abstract, spiritual families, social groups use of humans (roles in everyday life, connections to self, others and world)

Source: Printed with Dr. Lorraine Freedle's Permission.

The Neurosequential Model and Sandplay Therapy.

Freedle ©2019 (adapted from Perry ©2002–2019 and Damasio ©2010).

Freedle, I. R. "Making connections: Sandplay Therapy and the Neurosequential Model of Therapeutics," *Journal of Sandplay Therapy, 28*(1), 2019.

Sandplay's Neuro-Sensory Feedback Loop

© Freedle, 2006, 2007, 2019

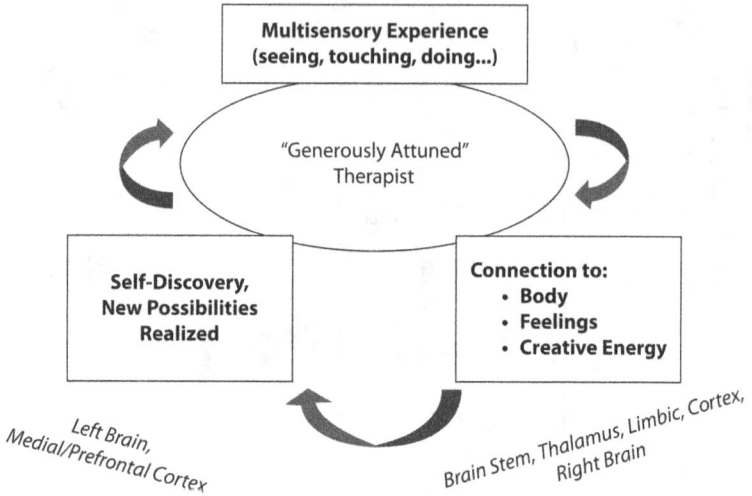

**Multisensory Experience
(seeing, touching, doing...)**

"Generously Attuned"
Therapist

**Self-Discovery,
New Possibilities
Realized**

Connection to:
- **Body**
- **Feelings**
- **Creative Energy**

*Left Brain,
Medial/Prefrontal Cortex*

*Brain Stem, Thalamus, Limbic, Cortex,
Right Brain*

Chart 8.1 Sandplay's Sensory Feedback Loop. Image by Dr. Lorraine Freedle

depressive and affective symptoms in the diencephalon. In the limbic section here, relational difficulties are located. I see this with many couples who are triggered by their partner.

Early childhood upsets and traumatic events are often held in the lower areas, the brainstem and diencephalon.

Many clients in IFSsandtray recall events for which they had no conscious memory. This is an example of implicit memory coming into consciousness. In years of practice, I have watched my clients' selecting figurines, often compelled for reasons their conscious mind cannot explain. When we begin to explore, we discover that the selection relates expressly to the Parts that hold the trauma. At this time evidence is anecdotal, but I have witnessed, and healed, clients who have experienced deep-seated trauma even before the age of five (see Chapter 9, *"Betty: Healing Early Childhood Trauma with the Pro-Symptom Belief Cards"*).

I ask these very young Parts to speak through the client's mouth; somehow, they can and do respond to my questions. This is despite the fact that they often are stuck at an age when they weren't able to use verbal language. The trauma, upsetting event, and core negative beliefs are somatically held in the Part's body. When I do an IFS technique called Direct Access, combined with a Sensorimotor technique that focuses on the sensations held within the body, the Part is able to feel sensations. I practice this technique to give Parts a voice to use where they didn't have one at such young ages when they are frozen at the time the upsetting or traumatic event occurred.

Training in a somatic therapy such as Sensorimotor Psychotherapy enables the practitioner to understand how the body holds trauma. In the book, *Sensorimotor Psychotherapy: Interventions for Trauma and Attachment* the author, Pat Ogden, writes,

> Becoming aware of body sensations opens up a whole new avenue of discovery for us, enriching our internal experience .... However, it can initially trigger emotions that feel out of control, especially after trauma. Your sensations may make you feel terrified, rageful, panicky, frustrated, inadequate, weak, or helpless.
>
> (2015, p. 200)

Dr. Richard Schwartz, founder of the Internal Family Systems modality, also believes, like me, that each Part has its own body and voice. In his book, *No Bad Parts: Healing Trauma & Restoring Wholeness with the Internal Family Systems Model*, He writes,

> Sometimes what you learn can be quite surprising. And for me, these emotions, sensations, thoughts, impulses, and other things are emanations from parts .... And, as you get to know that part, you will learn that it isn't just a thought, sensation, impulse, or emotion. Indeed, it will let you know that it has a whole range of feelings and thoughts, and it can tell you about the role it is in and why it does what it does.
>
> (2021 p. 26)

I trust in the techniques learned in Internal Family System, such as Direct Access, and Sensorimotor Psychotherapy modalities combined with the unconscious mind. In addition, I rely on the information I receive when the Parts retell their physically held sensations from upsetting events or traumas through focusing on their bodies.

Although I'd studied IFS, Sensorimotor psychotherapy, and Ericson hypnosis, the actual practice of observing the Parts led to a new understanding of how to work with them by focusing on the body of the Part(s) that hold trauma. When this happens, I see physical changes in the client's faces, bodies, and their tone of voice changes. This may seem like an extreme statement, and I believe most therapists working with Parts in this manner concur that they witness their clients physically transform, presenting tonal vocal changes and adjusted postures.

The second section of the chart is where the limbic system engages. The Polyvagal Theory and IFS training helps us to understand when the Parts are in sympathetic arousal. The clinical conditions listed are relational difficulties, alcohol, substance abuse, and I would add problematic sexual behavior, all known as Firefighters in IFS. This is the state in which individuals seeking treatment find themselves under duress as many of them are experiencing mental and sexual health issues.

Guilt and shame are located in the neocortex level of the brain as shown in Chart 8.1 I discuss Billy, a client who healed from his overwhelming struggle with sexual shame utilizing the modality of Kalffian Sandplay therapy (see Chapter 12)

Individuals who practice sandplay therapy move through a feedback loop of experience, access to emotions and sensations, reflection, and discovery (Freedle 2007, 2019). At this point, it is extremely important to recognize Freedle's research was based entirely on Kalffian sandplay. I have not found any research to date that reflects the same experience is happening in sandtray, but I imagine there may be some overlap. Chart 8.1 illustrates the multi-sensory experience that is occurring during a sandplay session.

In the center of the diagram sits the "Generously Attuned Therapist." Trained in Kalffian sandplay, the therapist understands the importance of silently witnessing the client from the moment they move around the room collecting their symbols/figurines. They place those miniatures in the tray, the therapist remaining quiet unless asked a specific question. In sandplay the therapist usually won't tell a client what to pick or any type of directive in a sandtray. The client learns no matter what they do, it's the right thing, ultimately learning they are also okay being themselves in the world. See Chapter 18 where my client Leona discusses this in her experience of both Kalffian Sandplay therapy and IFSsandtray.

At the top of the loop is neuroception, the five senses actively engaged in the process. The visceral aspects of playing in the sand—touching, manipulating, or even just picking up a miniature—are important activities that can trigger an internal response. That experience itself helps the client to connect to their own body. Frequently feelings emerge, and the right brain is activated. No words are needed at this point. The client's right brain is creatively solving the problem in the sandplay trays they are creating. The client then moves into the last section of the loop. At this stage, the therapist won't usually provide any interpretations. It is believed the client is experiencing a Self-Discovery, shown in the graphic, which emerges from their own system, as they discover new possibilities.

When a client begins to talk about upsetting events, they often become dysregulated, and sympathetically aroused. This engages the body's flight and fight response. When I see this happen, I immediately move into the sandplay room. I ask them to move the sand in the tray with their hands in any way that feels right to them. [I have included images of such trays. These trays were from clients who were dysregulated and calmed down within minutes. I think these trays are excellent examples of the feedback loop.]

Element of Tranquility: When Sand Regulates the Body and Calms the Mind

One particular client who I will call Cindy, arrived for her session completely dysregulated. Elaine, her partner of seven years, had recently broken up with her. They'd experienced many of these upheavals, always coming back together. This time, however, Cindy knew Elaine was serious and not going to change her mind. Cindy had been seeing me for problematic sexual behavior. She was going outside of her relationship and having sex with other people without obtaining Elaine's consent. This was a deal breaker for Elaine.

After a few minutes of talking, Cindy grew even more distressed, so I asked her to move into the sandplay room. Working with sand would help her come back into her body, allowing her to access a calmer state. I asked Cindy to begin by moving her hands in the sand. See Figure 8.1.

Within a few moments, her hands gently pushing the sand around. Cindy said, "This feels so wonderful. I wish I could put my feet in here."

It was then that I said, "Yes, let's do that. I have many other trays." I got up and moved a tray, placing it at Cindy's feet.

Cindy first touched the sand with her hands then put her feet in the tray and said, "This reminds me of my grandparent's house at the beach when I was young. I loved going to Maine to visit every summer. My grandmother always had my back, and I knew it." Cindy was now calm and able to stop crying. The sand had brought her back to an elemental time in her life; the tactile sensations reminded her of a time of freedom and peace. In this state of peace, she could better address what happened between herself and Elaine (Figure 8.2).

Another tray I wanted to share was made by my client Jane, whose healing I write about in Chapters 13 and 14. In one session she arrived at the session in an agitated state, her jaw clenched, and shoulders hunched, the result of a sympathetically charged autonomic nervous system. We immediately moved into the sandplay room where I asked her to move her hands in the

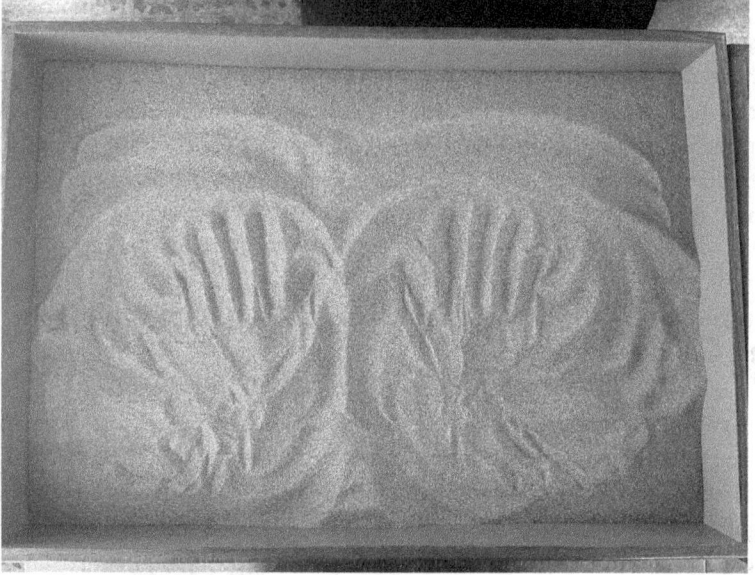

Figure 8.1 Cindy's Tray of Moving the Sand with Her Hands

Photo by the author

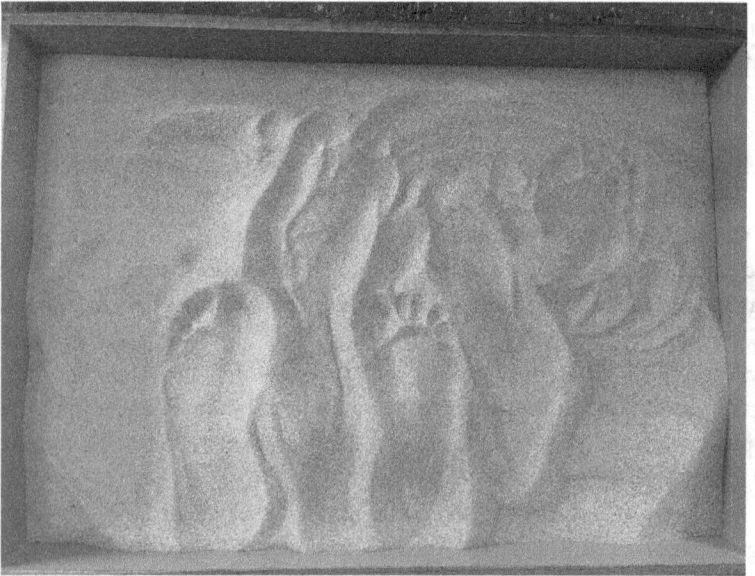

Figure 8.2 Cindy's Footprints in the Sand

Photo by the author

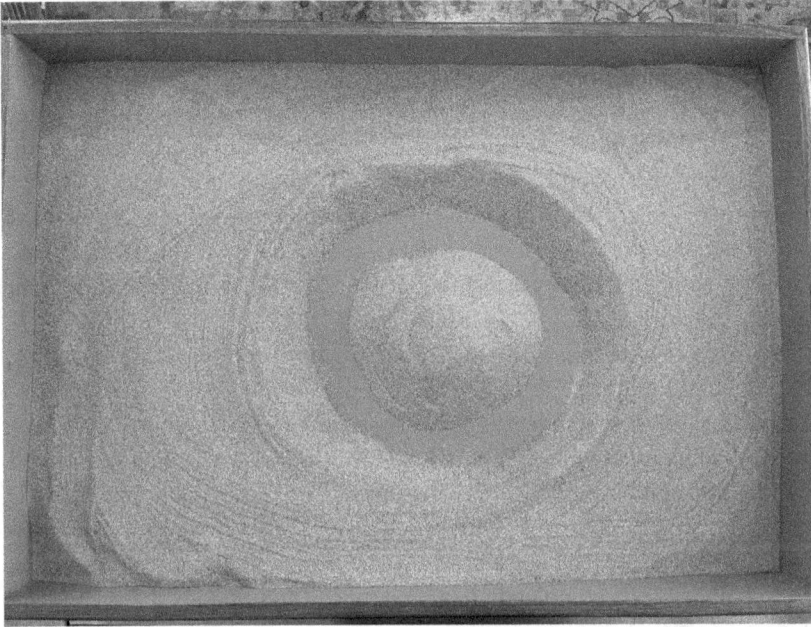

Figure 8.3 Jane's Calming Circle

Photo by the author.

tray of sand. See Figure 8.3 for the photograph of what her tray looked like when she finished.

To me this image is symbolic just by itself. I'm often excited when I witness one of my clients create a circular image in the sand. It is almost spiritual when someone begins to make circles or spirals in the sand, often a circular image in sandplay can be thought of as a Self-symbol one of wholeness. A sense of wholeness often brings an internal sense of calmness and clarity which is ventral vagal in the Polyvagal Theory. A spiral can be sometimes thought of as a client going deeper into the unconscious or coming out of the depths of the unconscious.

At first when Jane sat before the sand tray, she was so dysregulated she was trembling. I asked her to get comfortable, by either standing up or sitting in the chair. She said she preferred sitting, reaching both arms over the sand, and placing her right hand into her left palm, making a tight fist. It took her to just take a few minutes to place her hands into the sand. She began moving both hands together in a fast, jerky manner without any perceivable rhythm. The sand almost spilled out of the container of the tray, it moved from one side to the other. and Jane grew teary. After a few minutes, she slowed the movement and began making circular movements with her hands around the whole tray. There were approximately three inches of loosely packed sand under her moving hands.

She worked the sand until a mound rose almost exactly from the center, slightly to the right. Next, she used the palm of her hands to flatten the sand outside the mound. She then began moving the mound in a circular motion, creating a flat ring or disc. Her breathing was slowing down and she looked like she was in a trance state—it didn't appear she could see me. I quietly witnessed her eyes follow her hands, moving the top of the sand around the mound.

Within a few moments she took three of her forefingers and began moving the sand beside the four-inch mound of sand she made. The dry sand would slide down where her fingers just cleared it, exposing the blue base of the tray. The exposed blue began to look like a moat surrounding the mound. She then reached over to a cart to her left where I keep water, hand towels, and various types of brushes on a cart. She grabbed a three-inch paintbrush and began using it to move the sand. At that moment I became very curious. I watched her body completely relax. I recalled Cindy's body doing the same thing when she placed her feet in the tray.

As I watched, Jane moved from a sympathetic dysregulated state and shifted into a calm ventral vagal state within five minutes, maybe less. She began clearing all the sand grains from the blue circle with the side of the one-inch-wide brush. At this point, Jane struggled with the dry sand. It slid down from the sides into the clear blue moat she was creating. I wondered how she was going to handle this aspect of working with dry sand. Was it going to dysregulate her out of frustration? I waited, trusting my client's unconscious in this process.

She reached over to the cart again and selected a one-inch soft makeup brush out of the many brushes placed in a small cart at the end of the tray. Many of my clients use this brush when working in the sand because of its fine bristles. These fine hairs move sand particles easily to expose a clear blue base.

Now her movements became fluid, like creating a painting. She instinctively knew where all the brushes were located, as if she had used them before, despite the fact she never had used any items on the cart before. I believe her unconscious knew exactly where everything in the room was located including the brushes; she had passed that cart numerous times before.

With tremendous dexterity, she used the one-inch brush like an experienced artist who knows how to use a palette knife to put oil paint on a canvas.

Many artists know this creative space well. Jane now used the smaller brush inside the blue circle and moved around that circle five times or more. With each sweep of the brush, she moved the fallen particles of sand to the sides, one by one. Something truly amazing was happening; she was becoming one with the process.

Selecting the three-inch paint brush, she worked the outside of the blue circle, creating a pattern at the top. Satisfied, she picked up the one-inch brush again to make sure that exposed blue was absolutely without one speck of sand. She lifted her head, looked into my eyes, and calmly asked, "What the hell was that?" She paused, looked at the tray again, and then added, "Can you believe what just happened? I am so calm now."

I nodded my head. "I know it's unbelievable how that happens" and we just looked at each other silently with a sense of awe.

So many of my clients' experiences, like both Cindy and Jane's, have convinced me how the Sandplay Sensory Feedback Loop works when anyone who is feeling dysregulated works in the sand. So many of my clients—working without words, without explanation—experience this same shift, experiencing a profound sense of healing, sometimes in minutes. Sandplay has the power to calm the autonomic nervous system, bring curiosity, and Self-connection to the client.

Freedle's Sandplay's Neuro-Sensory Feedback Loop discussed earlier in this chapter, brings the client into the multisensory experience which connects them to their body, feelings, and creative energy. And at the same time, stimulating the sections of the right brain including the brain stem, thalamus, and the limbic cortex. Followed by the client having new Self-discoveries, realizing new possibilities, and then stimulating the left-brain areas such as the medial/prefrontal cortex.

References

Freedle, L. R. "Sandplay therapy with brain injured adults: An exploratory qualitative study," *Journal of Sandplay Therapy*, 16(2), 2007, pp. 115–133.

Freedle, L. R. "Making connections: Sandplay therapy and the neurosequential model of therapeutics," *Journal of Sandplay Therapy*, 28(1), 2019, pp. 91–109.

Freud, S. *On dreams*. Translated by M. D. Eder. Digireads.com Publishing, New York, NY, 2019/1901. ISBN 13:-1-4209-6527-5.

Jung, C. J. *Man and his symbols*. Dell Publishing, New York, NY, 1964 (p. 220).

Ogden, P., *Sensorimotor psychotherapy: Interventions for trauma and attachment*. W.W. Norton & Company, New York, NY, 2015 (p. 200).

Schwartz, R., *No bad parts: Healing trauma & restoring wholeness with the internal family systems model.* Sounds True, Boulder, CO, 2021 (p. 26).

Wiersma, J. K., Freedle, L. R., McRoberts, R., & Solberg, K., "A meta-analysis of sandplay therapy treatment outcomes," *International Journal of Play Therapy*, 31(4), 2022, pp. 197–215. https://doi.org/10.1037/pla0000180

Section Two

Courageous Souls Who Heal with In-Depth Therapy

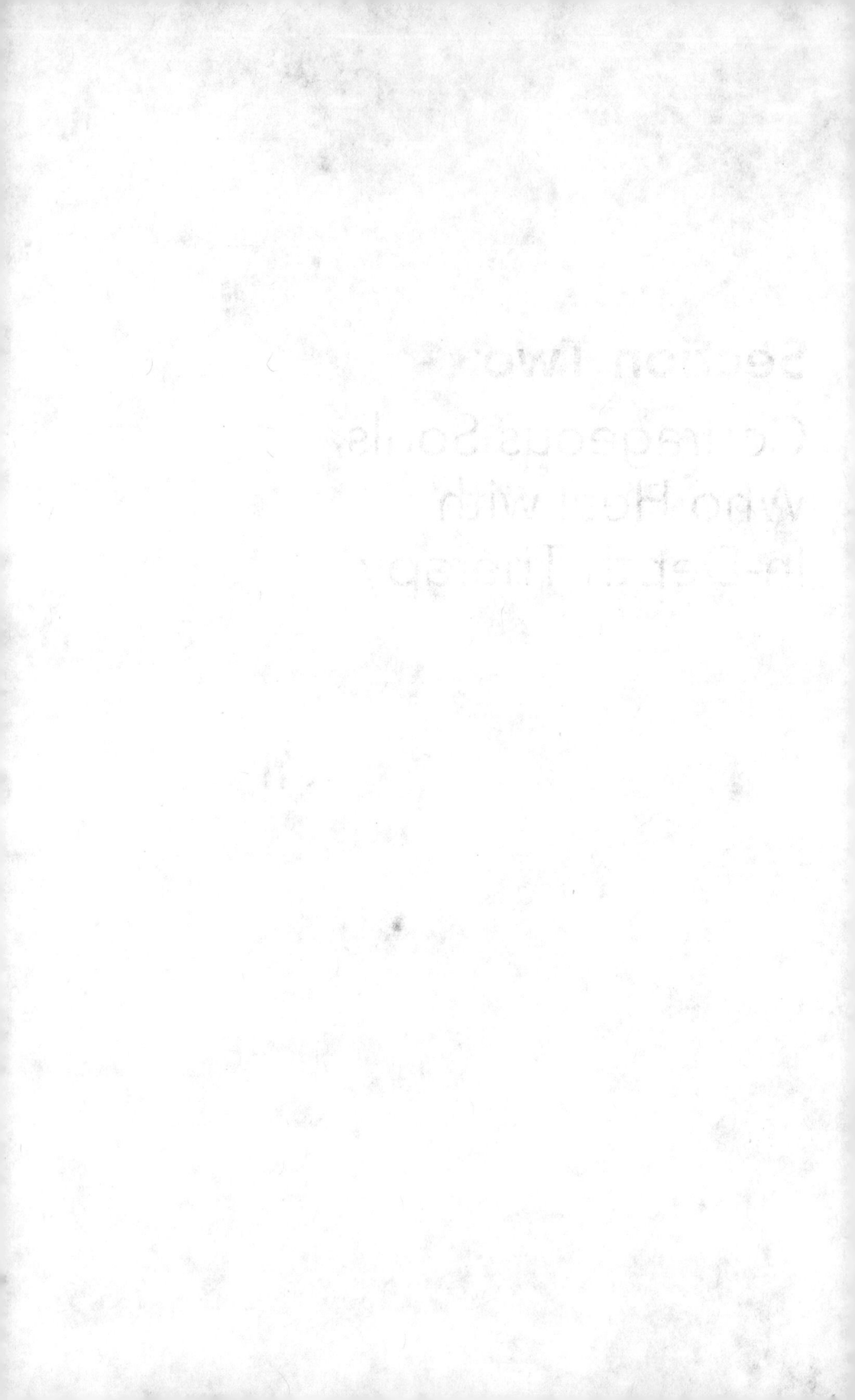

Betty   9

Healing Early Childhood
Trauma with the
Pro-Symptom Belief Cards

As a doctor who specializes in several different forms of treatment, my intention is to find the right modality that best suits the client. Many of my choices are intuitive and informed by my deep understanding of the effectiveness of alternative means of treatment. This chapter focuses on one client, sharing one session in which we did not use sand and miniatures to access the subconscious. Instead, we used something I designed, Pro-Symptom Belief Cards (PSBC). These cards, each with a saying corresponding to deeply held feelings, allow me to better understand what limiting thoughts or ideas might be blocking clients from healing. (For a detailed explanation of the cards and their application, see Chapter 15.)

Before I ever invite clients to dig their fingers into the sand, or select miniatures, we begin with talk. As stated before, talk therapy is important, especially when used in conjunction with other techniques. In the following case, talk therapy led us to a greater understanding of the problems. When it feels right, I introduce the PSBC to take us further.

But, as illustrated in this session, I don't depend on the Pro-Symptom Belief Cards alone to address my client's needs. My training in Internal Family Systems, Sensorimotor Psychotherapy, and Hypnotherapy comes into play, as well as many years of observing and understanding nonverbal communication. The cards, in this case, allow me to use cross-disciplinary techniques to address the issues at hand.

Betty, a pseudonym, entered treatment with me after 15 years of working with therapists who all utilized various forms of talk therapy. Betty didn't feel

DOI: 10.4324/9781003388302-11

it was helping her and was looking for something different. She found my website and contacted me. After speaking with her for only a few minutes, it was obvious to me Betty had experienced early childhood trauma which had affected her both emotionally and physically. She informed me at that time she was also under the care of a few medical specialists who were testing for several physical disorders, but all the results so far had been negative, leaving her doctors perplexed. I immediately thought of what Dr. Stephen Porges called Medically Unexplained Symptoms (MUS) and I thought this was happening to Betty.

Betty is a 65-year-old heterosexual woman who has been married, divorced, and now partnered with Jerome. They have been together for 4 years, and 1 year earlier Jerome moved into Betty's home. He doesn't have children, is retired, and believes in doing the right thing. Betty is the fourth child born into a family with eight children, an alcoholic father who had anger issues, and a caring mother. Both of her parents are deceased. Her father was self-employed as a mechanic, couldn't support the family on his income, and her mother worked at a manufacturing plant from 3:30 in the afternoon to 11:30 at night.

Due to her parent's financial insecurity, her mother's hours, and an emotionally unavailable father, she took a major role in caretaking for her younger siblings when she was in her mid-teens. Betty had to plan dinners, cook them, and watch over her younger siblings while they did their homework. When she came to me, she was unable to maintain a job due to physical illnesses and was on a limited income.

Betty had one child, Jenny, who died from a heroin overdose at the age of twenty-four. Betty was forty when she passed away. Jenny had three children, her first child was adopted as an infant, and she raised the other two. Unfortunately, when Jenny died, her oldest was only four and the younger child was three. Upon Jenny's death, these two children were placed in Betty's care.

We were working together for six weeks when the following session occurred. On that day Betty emailed me earlier in the week and said she did have one particular issue she wanted to work on in her next session. So, I placed the Pro-Symptom Belief Cards on the table next to where she normally sat. She arrived, took her seat, spent a few minutes checking in, and she said she still wanted to work on the problem she emailed me about.

What you are about to read has been transcribed from the actual session, which was completed in approximately thirty-eight minutes. For the sake of expediency, I have edited out repetition when it didn't further the narrative function—edits will be indicated by an ellipsis in brackets [...]. Throughout I have abbreviated my name to the initial P, and Betty to B.

The Session started at 3:14 pm

When we started, Betty's face was drawn, tight, and she appeared physically and emotionally stressed.

P: So, you have an issue you came in with today, tell me what that is.

B: Well, the issue I have are my two grandchildren, who are young adults and are twenty-two and twenty-three. Both children are needing assistance and are now moving back home. Jerome thinks we should all eat dinner together as a family. I am trying to get him to understand they are young adults and need to live their own lives.

In this instance it's important to confirm what I heard.

P: Yes, so there's an issue where you have difficulty talking to Jerome about this?

B: Yes.

P: Alright, so, I have placed a deck of cards next to you they are called Pro-Symptom Belief Cards. I want you to look at them and whatever you feel is true for you when you think about telling him the kids are older and they're not going to sit as a family. Put the cards you don't feel are true about yourself in another pile.

Betty takes about one and a half minutes to put the cards into two piles.

B: Okay, I have picked three cards.

P: Okay, what are they?

B: One is "I am not good enough," the other is "I feel inadequate," and "I am permanently damaged."

P: Out of the three, which one feels like, "yeah, this is it in my body," You feel a sensation in your body, and you just feel it's more true than the others?

B: Okay

P: Which one is it?

B: "I am inadequate."

P: So, what I want you to do is put them all on the table beside you.

Betty gathers up the cards and places them on the table beside her.

P: So, what I want you to do now, is just focus in a moment, and I am going to have you close your eyes.

[This was the second session in which we worked with these cards; Betty was familiar with the process] *Betty has closed her eyes. I say the following to put her at ease.*

P: If you don't want to close your eyes then look at a point in the wall behind me, but I see you closed your eyes, that's great. The reason I have you close your eyes is that I want you to focus on the internal sensations and feelings in your body. Think of the issue of telling your boyfriend that you don't think it's going to happen. You don't think the kids are going to want to eat dinner at the same time. And you feel the words "I'm inadequate," focus on the sensations you feel in your body, like you might have something in your throat or stomach or chest. Just focus on the sensations inside your body, and as you focus on the sensations … do you have one now? Do you feel something in your body?

B: Yes, my chest feels a little heavy.

P: Yes, as your chest feels heavy, how heavy does it feel? Like a one pound, two pound or elephant's foot? What's the weight on your chest?

B: Maybe just a pound.

P: Alright, what I want you to do is focus on the scene of talking with your boyfriend, with the words "I'm inadequate." Focus on that heavy chest feeling, that one-pound weight and as you focus on that one-pound weight, just notice the weight on the chest, that one-pound weight on your chest, the heavy weight on your chest and the words "I'm inadequate." And see when you felt the same identical heaviness in your chest, and I know you are sixty-five, before sixty-five "Focus on that same heavy chest feeling before sixty-five. Just let the body show you, there might be a scene or an image, let something come up."

I pause and wait for a few seconds. I allow my voice to take on a slow, hypnotic tone, and my words are very deliberate, a style derived directly from my hypnosis training.

B: I just feel like in my teenage years, maybe about seventeen or eighteen.

P: Yes, is there a scene that comes up around seventeen or eighteen?

B: Yeah, I was a wild one, I ran a little wild. So, I just feel the heaviness on my chest because I did some crazy things.

P: Yes, was there a scene that came up when you were seventeen years or eighteen years old when you felt the heaviness. Is there a particular scene that shows up when you were in your late teens? When you actually felt that same identical heaviness. Focus on the heaviness alone, as if that's the only thing you have to focus on now. Do you feel that sensation of heaviness? What was the scene you were in when you felt the same heaviness when you were being the wild one. "What's the scene that pops up?"

B: Just having sex with someone.

P: Excellent. Sex with someone, yes. So, as you're having sex with someone do you see the image now of having sex with this person?

B: Yes.

P: As you see the scene of having sex with this person, what's the feeling in your body as if you were seventeen now as you are having sex with this person? Focus on having sex with this person focus on your body then as if it is happening now. Be in your seventeen-year-old body as if it's now and now is then, just focus on that heaviness in your chest, see if there are any other sensations that you're feeling as you're having sex with this other person.

B: "No, I wouldn't say I have another sensation. Well, it is a sensation, I was brought up Catholic, so I was always taught it was wrong to have sex before you were married."

P: Yes, I want you to think about that scene now. As you're having sex and maybe feeling it's wrong, because it felt wrong.

B: Yes.

P: So, what I want you to focus on is what it felt like at that time when it felt wrong. Just focus on when it felt it was wrong to have sex before you were married.

B: Yes, it was wrong, and my stomach felt a little upset.

P: Stomach was upset. Is there another sensation than the stomach is upset, was that the only one?

B: No, just my chest and my body. It puts a burden on you.

P: "Yes, it's a burden. So, what I want you to focus on now is the burden. As if you are in the scene now having sex and feeling this burden in your chest and the upset stomach do you feel it now as if now was then?"

The phrase "… now is then and then is now" is akin to the confusion technique learned in hypnosis trainings, which allows the client to access the unconscious.

B: Hmmm, No.

P: So, what I want you to focus on now is being in that scene, as if you're in that scene now, as if you're seventeen now, like now is then and then is now, does that make sense?

P: Yes.

P: As you are seventeen now, focus on that scene having sex and notice your stomach is upset. What are the sensations in the stomach?

B: Ahh, like jumpy.

P: Yes, as it's jumpy, can you describe the sensations of jumpy?

B: Well, it's more like a nervous energy.

P: Yes.

B: It just feels like it's kind of grumbling.

P: Okay, it's kind of like a grumbling feeling?

B: Yes.

P: So, do you still feel that heaviness in your chest?

B: Well, I feel it more on the heart right now.

P: Yes, what's happening on the heart?

B: It's beating very, very, fast.

P: So, it's really rapidly beating.

B: Yes

P: I want you to focus on this rapidly beating heart and this nervous grumbling feeling in your tummy. Focus on those two together as if that's the only thing you have to do now. You're seventeen now with that rapidly beating heart with a nervous grumbly feeling in your tummy. When did you feel those two sensations?

B: I would say about fifteen.

P: As you are fifteen, what's the scene that popped up?

B: Having to take care of my siblings.

P: Yes, as you are having to take care of your siblings. Just notice what you are feeling in your body. What's the scene you are in now as you are having to take care of your siblings.

B: I am envisioning having to be home, cleaning the house, picking up, and gotta make supper for everybody. Trying to help everybody with their homework. It's just a lot. You're always moving, my heart beating 'cause you have to run around, my stomach is upset 'cause I am being pulled in different directions. That's what I feel like.

P: Yes, I want you to focus now as you are in that scene, running around, making dinner, cleaning the house, and helping other kids with their homework. Focus on that fast-beating heart at the same time as the upset stomach. When did you feel that before fifteen?

B: Hmmm, I would say when I was about ten.

P: What happened in the scene at ten?

B: Well, my mother did not tell us the facts of life, or me anyhow. Then I became a young woman, and I really did not know what was happening to me.

P: Are you saying when you got your period?

B: Yes.

P: Okay, as you got your period what was happening where were you?

B: I was in the bathroom downstairs.

P: Yes, as you were in the bathroom downstairs, focus on that scene as if now is then and then is now when you got your period, you didn't know what was going on when you got your period, is that right?

B: Yes.

P: Focus that scene now as you are ten. Focus on the sensations in your body when you got your period.

B: I was very scared, crying a little bit because I thought something was wrong with me. So, that's how I felt.

P: Yes, focus on that scared feeling. What do you notice in your body as you are feeling scared in that moment thinking something is wrong with you. Focus on scared.

B: All over my body. I was shaking, crying, and sadness.

P: Yes, I want you to focus on your body being scared, shaking, crying, and being sad. Focus on shaking and crying. See when you felt that before ten years old.

B: I would say probably when I was about three.

I started working this way a few years ago and found clients, when asked to concentrate on their bodily sensations. These sensations can often connect to things that happen before the age of five. I discovered this accidently, tried it with numerous clients over the years, began trusting my instincts, and integrated various modalities. Frequently, clients would find themselves experiencing younger and younger memories when absorbed in the qualities of the sensations in their bodies. Now I know if clients are able to connect with their body, they will be candidates for healing with this therapeutic method.

Usually, in the beginning of treatment—within the first two or three sessions—I will test this out by asking them to look at the Pro-Symptom Belief Cards, find which ones fit when they think about the very issues they are experiencing. Often if they can't drop deeper into the sensations, this is usually because they are disconnected from their bodies. With these individuals I know sandplay is where I will start the therapeutic process with them.

P: Yes, what happened at three? What's the scene you see now?

B: Well, I see my brother cutting my favorite doll's head off with a meat cutter. He's cutting the doll's head off. So, I was very sad.

P: So, he took the doll and put it in a meat cutter and cut the head off?

B: Yes.

P: Did you see that?

B: Yes, I did see that.

P: You saw that, so you're in the scene where you see your brother cut your doll's head off with a meat cutter; focus on that and as your three now just watching that scene focus on what's happening in your body as you see your favorite doll's head being cut off.

B: Yes, I am very mad, angry, and upset.

P: Yes, how do you feel mad, angry, and also upset in your body? How did that show up as a sensation?

B: As a sensation I, actually umm … it feels real hard, like you want to hit or stomp on something.

P: Yes. Focus on your feeling like you want to stomp on something and how did you feel that upset? Did you feel it that mad wanting to hit, stomp, or punch something, and you felt that in your feet? Is that right?

B: Yes.

P: Yes, focus on when you want to stomp on something, you're upset, and want to punch something. Just focus on you're so upset, mad and angry, you want to stomp on something, and punch something. Is that right?

B: Yes. Well, my brother cut his thumb at the time. I was also very scared for him and nervous. We ran into the house.

P: Focus on that. Running into the house. What's the scene when you run into the house?

B: Well, I was scared and my mother had to take him to the hospital. I was upset because he cut the doll's head off and he was getting all the attention. No one was listening to me and I was sad, crying and upset, and I had no comforting.

P: Yes, so you were sad, crying and upset, and not getting comforted, focus on that. As your brother is being taken care of and you're sad, crying, and upset. Focus on that now and what's the sensations in the body?

B: Mm, I have tears as I am crying, upset, mad, but they're all physical things I want to do at this point because I am just sitting aside and my body goes limp.

P: As your body goes limp. When did you go limp before three, when you felt the same limp feeling or was this the first time?

Asking that last question: "is this the first time?" is critical because that will determine if it goes younger than three. I have had clients answer no at this time and will go back earlier in life.

B: No, this was the first time.

I can now begin healing all the Parts which were frozen in time, in her implicit memory held in the body by sensations. I believe this is tied into what Dr. Stephen Porges labeled neuroception. These sensations are held in the Part's body and are held with the Pro-Symptom Belief. For Betty that began with "I am inadequate." At the time of each of these upsetting events, Betty's system held the sensations which can be accessed as you have just read above. I then can use the techniques I integrated and go back to each Part that was frozen in time. It's critical to go to the first memory, especially those held in the implicit mind, before the age of four or five. The session continues.

P: As this was the first time, would you like to have an experience of healing from this?

B: Yes

P: Okay, what I want you to do is focus on being three and being limp, do you want to let that go to the earth, air, water, fire, spirit, or something else?

Letting go to the elements is used in the unburdening stage in Internal Family Systems. The Parts, when accessed somatically, this very young Part known as the Exile, will let go of the burdens it holds in its body.

B: Umph, fire.

P: "Let it go to the fire now, I want you to imagine a fire, and let go of that limp feeling that anger, sadness, terrible feelings, and all of that, and let me know when it's done."

B: (after a long pause) It's done.

P: Great! As you let go …

Betty is now smiling and begins to laugh. I have no idea why, so I ask,

P: What's so funny?

B: Well, it's going up there. Out of the body.

P: Yes, is it all gone or is it still going?

B: Yes, it's all gone

P: As it's all gone, do you want to have a new quality? What quality would you like to have? As you're three and let go to the fire, ask the three-year-old what quality she would want.

B: Yes.

P: Ask her what quality she would like to have as you see her in your mind's eye. Ask her.

B: (to herself) What quality would you like to have? I think it's speaking up for herself.

P: Did she say that, or did you say that? Ask her what she would like.

B: Well, she wants some attention.

P: Yes, ask her who she wants some attention from.

B: She wants attention from her mother.

P: Okay, can her mother give her attention now

B: No, her mother can't give her attention because she is too busy with the brother that cut his thumb.

P: Yes, I am wondering. Can you give her attention now? The adult you?

B: Yes, I can give her a lot of attention.

P: Yes, give her from your adult self now, attention to the three-year-old.

Betty waves her left arm to the side, curls it at the elbow, and brings her arm back to her stomach area, and says out loud.

B: Come here honey. Let me hug you. What's going on with you?

B: (mimicking a child's voice) My doll's head was cut off and nobody cares.

She opens her eyes and looks directly at me.

P: Just go with that.

Betty closes her eyes immediately and puts her head back and rests it on the back of sofa.

P: Let her show you how upset she is. Tell me when she is done showing you.

B: (after a pause) She's done

P: Ask her if she thinks you got her pain.

B: Do you think I got your pain now? ... She said 'no.'

P: Ask her what you didn't get.

B: What did I not get? She says you actually took all my pain away.

P: Yes, ask her if she wants to let go of the pain to the fire.

B: She said yes.

P: Great. Have her do that now.

B: Okay, let it go (to the three-year-old) Okay, she let it go.

P: Ask her now, what quality she would like that she didn't get from her mother or anyone else. What quality would she like to get.

B: "What quality would you like to get, that you didn't get from your mother (pause) I think she wants the quality that she will be able to speak on her behalf and people will listen to her."

P: Yes, ask her.

It's important to listen carefully. When a client says "I think" they are getting the information not from the three-year-old, but by thinking.

B: Okay, three-year-old, who are you going to get that quality from (pause) She really doesn't know.

As I hear this, I realized this three-year-old had Parts of herself which don't know, but when I reframe the question, another Part will know.

P: Ask her if she did know where she could get that quality from, ask the Part of her that doesn't know to step back, and ask her if she knows now if she knows if she can get that quality now, who speaks up?

Parts having Parts is taught in the Internal Family Systems trainings. Knowing this I asked the Part of the three-year-old that didn't know to step back, let the Part that knows to answer, and it did. (For more information on Parts see Chapter 5.)

B: Her grandmother.

P: Yes, ask her if her grandmother can give her that quality to her now.

B: Yes, she said yes.

P: Ask her can she get it from her grandmother now?

B: Yes.

P: So, ask her to get that quality of speaking up from the grandmother now.

B: Okay. Can you get if from your grandmother? (Pause) Yes

P: Yes, have her get that quality of speaking up from the grandmother. Tell me when she is done.

B: She's done.

P: Great, ask her does she want to leave that scene, or be a different age than three? This is just for her.

B: She said, yes, she wants to leave that scene.

P: Ask her where she wants to go.

B: She wants to be older.

P: Ask her how old she wants to be?

B: She said twenty-one.

P: Ask her where she wants to be twenty-one now. Ask her where she wants to try being twenty-one now.

B: She wants to be in her own apartment being self-sufficient.

P: Yes, ask her to find an apartment, see what she needs to be self-sufficient, and ask her to tell you what that is. See if she can try that out now and ask her does she need anything as she is now twenty-one in her apartment.

B: Oh, well she said she needs to get a job, and she has to look in the ads in the paper.

She paused for a few seconds. [Betty was in connection with the Part, this is a desired response in IFS, and known as a Self to Part connection. Self has many "C" qualities such as compassion, curiosity, clarity, etc. ... When a client is coming from Self and is in relationship to the Part, Parts will change and know what they want to do].

B: Okay, she found an apartment.

P: Great, does she need anything now that she has found an apartment?

B: Yes, she needs to furnish it.

P: Yes, have her furnish it now.

B: Okay, it's furnished.

P: Okay ask her does she need anything else.

B: Well, she needs a job.

P: Tell her to find a job.

B: Well, she's actually working a job, but she needs more hours.

P: Okay, tell her to speak up and get more hours.

B: Okay, she asked her boss, now it's good. (laughing)

P: Okay, does it feel complete, or does she need something else?

B: No, she said it's complete.

Throughout the remainder of the session, we continue along this vain, checking in with Betty at different ages where she was stuck, ascertaining the security the wounded Parts need, and healing all of them just like the three year old.

When we ended the session, Betty was smiling, her eyes twinkling, and she no longer believed she was inadequate. She said, "I now know what to say to Jerome, how to handle the situation, and my body feels relaxed, and I am feeling calm inside."

The Session stopped at 3:53 pm

Utilizing this technique with clients is helpful, and effective, and often heals clients from core negative self-concepts within one session as shown in this session with Betty. It is especially helpful for clinicians who don't work with sand and miniatures. Utilizing the PSBC combined accessing the body somatically, and knowledge of how Parts can be effective in healing individuals with early childhood wounds.

When working with individuals who have Parts that are scared, resistant, anxious, or any other concerns the client may inform the clinician they don't want to do this experiential exercise. This is reasonable and in that situation, the clinician can check in with their own Parts. Are they confident about this process or do they find themselves questioning the validity of using the PSBC, anxious in any way, or insecure about their own abilities to engage in experiential learning? Once the clinician has checked with their own Parts and is confident, they can and should try the experiential exercise with their clients. Whenever the client's Parts have questions or concerns and they are answered the Parts may relax allowing the experiential to happen. Even skeptical Parts will engage if their concerns are addressed.

Going back into the implicit memory, often before the age of five, is critical in healing because humans' brains form from the brainstem up as shown in Chapter 7, "What Goes in the Backpack? The Four B's: Beliefs, Body, Brain, and Behavior. The Neurosequential Model of Therapeutics (NMT), designed by Dr. Bruce Perry, is significant and essential to comprehending early childhood trauma, and how these formative years are just a baseline of how the brain will develop into adulthood.

In the 2009 issue of the *Journal of Loss and Trauma*, Perry writes,

> … the malleability of the brain shifts during development, and there for the timing and specific 'pattern' of neglect influence the final functional outcome. A child deprived of consistent, attentive, and attuned nurturing for the first 3 years of life who is then adopted and begins to receive attention, love, and nurturing may not be capable of benefiting from these experiences with the same malleability as an infant. In some cases, this later love is insufficient to overcome the dysfunctional organization of the neural systems mediating socioemotional interactions.

When in-depth treatments are used such as in the case of Betty using the PSBC or sandplay, individuals can heal from early childhood trauma because their brains develop new neuropathways. See Chapter 15 to learn more about working with the PSBC.

Resource

Perry, B., "Examining childhood maltreatment through a neurodevelopmental lens: Clinical applications of the neurosequential model of therapeutics," *Journal of Loss and Trauma*, 2009. https://doi.org/10.1080/15325020903004350

Billy

10

Head Down, Holding Shameful Secrets

When I met Billy, a pseudonym, for the first time I opened my office door to the waiting room, feeling abruptly astonished, and taken aback by my internal perceptions. For a second, this man reminded me of a famous actor I'd often admired. He was dressed in dark jeans, a blue button-down dress shirt, brown leather loafers, and a lambskin leather jacket. I felt drawn to this tall handsome man with an athletic build, dark hair, and a soft engaging smile. I liked his sense of style.

Details of a person matter to me, and I make note of all of them. I think this attention to a person's body is due to the many years of wide-ranging training I have taken, especially the Polyvagal Theory and Sensorimotor Psychotherapy. These techniques taught me to notice minute aspects when a person takes a deep breath, sighs, swallows, does or doesn't make eye contact, twitches, and many other movements. I also learned to pay attention to my own bodily responses when I find myself with a pit in my stomach or some other sensation.

A week earlier, over the phone, Billy had asked about my professional services, my training in sex therapy that specialized in treating out of control sexual behavior (OCSB). I invited him to the room where I meet clients. We began talking. Billy told me how his life was everything he'd ever dreamed yet he was holding a *dangerous* secret—a secret that, if it got out, would cost him his marriage, his happiness, and the loss of his beloved partner, his wife, Regina. I immediately was curious about what he was holding so close to the vest and not able to tell her?

We continued the intake interview; he shared with me many of the wonderful qualities he found in Regina: she was intelligent, athletic, and stoic. I noticed

DOI: 10.4324/9781003388302-12

his eyes softened. He spoke about how much they loved being and playing together. They would frequently travel to exotic places where they would enjoy outdoor activities and amazing adventures. Billy said, "I never thought I wanted kids, and Regina has a daughter, Janet who has three children. I love Janet and those three little kids who all call me Grampy." He reached over to grab a tissue and began to tear up. "I love being a grandfather. I never thought I would want grandchildren; I adore those children. I can't bear the thought of not having them in my life if something happens between Regina and me." I noticed myself sinking deeper into Billy's story.

Billy wiped away his tears, took a deep breath, and looked at me. "She is the best scuba partner anyone could have. You know I have over three hundred dives under my belt, and Regina holds her own." His eyes and voice changed slightly in that moment as he talked about their last scuba vacation. It was as if, for a minute, he was back in his body, with a sense of pride about himself, and his relationship with Regina.

I thought to myself, with the irony of metaphor: "Oh, you think you have deep dives under your scuba belt? Wait until you dive into your depths of your unconscious with sandplay."

I brought my attention back to his voice which was now deeper and filled with sadness as he said, "I never in my wildest dreams believed I was capable of marrying anyone. I dated hundreds of women, and I once believed that under no circumstances would I ever consider a serious committed relationship." Internally I jumped when he abruptly added, "I am so ashamed of myself. I love my wife and I don't know how I can ever tell her what I've done. I know Regina will divorce me and I will lose my grandchildren." I listened to him tell me this, and took a deep breath, wondering what he could have done that was so terrible. As I watched him sitting with his head in his hands, I was touched with compassion. He lingered for a long time before he looked up at me.

I asked if he could share a little about his childhood. He began talking about an experience he had with a group of teens, and he was only around the age of five. The teenage boys told him to give each of them oral sex, which he did. A young child, Billy didn't understand why the teens wouldn't give him oral sex when it was his turn. He remembered hearing his mother calling for him and the boys stopped. Billy ran home and when his mother saw him, she yelled, "Why is your zipper down? What's wrong with you?" The adult Billy sitting in front of me said, "I was mortified, couldn't speak to her, I felt embarrassed and disgraced. I don't ever think I will forget disappointing her at that moment."

He was giving me all this information; I watched him move his head up out of his hands and looked away from me. He wiped away the tears gently streaming down his face with the back of his hand. I listened carefully and thought to myself, "I wonder if he can see any correlation of his distress of telling his wife his secret with the unpleasant feelings of letting his mother down." I waited a few more moments until he again made eye contact with me, and I gently asked, "I wonder if there was anything else you would like to share?"

Billy discussed being circumcised at the age of three. For some unknown reason, he woke up while it was happening, remembered being terrified, and said the circumcision failed. "I asked him how this was even possible." He had no idea how that happened or why his parents were having the procedure done. He was raised Catholic. He couldn't comment any further about it.

He recalled when he was around nine years old, he was bullied at school, and the other kids made fun of him. When I prompted him to tell me more about what that was like for him, he replied, "Yeah, it was a hard time and I got them back. I started working out, and I kicked the shit out of each of them. They never bothered me again."

He continued, "when I was eleven or twelve, we moved into a new house. I was exploring the basement where the furnace was located, and there was another section where there was a small makeshift room. The previous owner was a photographer and used this area to develop his pictures. The edges of the wall were separating, and I said to myself I wonder what was behind the barrier. I pulled a corner and saw what was hidden. It was a treasure trove, loaded with *Playboy*, *Penthouse*, other sexual magazines, and some raw photographs of naked women I think he must have taken." He reminded me of his age now, being close to sixty years old, and said, "You have to remember this was long before the internet and some of those pictures shocked me." I asked him to describe what he saw. "I just remember the magazines were nothing compared to the photos. These explicit pictures depicted titillating women with thin bodies and big tits. I found them to be super sexy. The women posed in awkward positions, with their legs spread eagle. I got turned on when I looked at them." He paused for a moment, and said, "that's about it for my childhood."

"I then asked," "is there anything I didn't ask that you might like me to know?"

"Oh yeah, I remember my first girlfriend I fell in love with when I was eighteen. She dumped me when I asked her if she ever thought about anal play. She said I was disgusting, and I felt huge amounts of shame for having asked. I was heartbroken and so upset about her leaving me. I felt horrible. I think I had even more shame because my father thought men who were gay were vulgar'."

I was wondering if he still was struggling with his devastating emotions from his past including the feeling of disappointing his mother, and the loss of his first girlfriend. I speculated this might have to do with what was related to the very secret that he felt was going to end the life he loved with Regina.

I asked him if he and Regina ever engaged in anal play and he responded, "absolutely not. She thinks it's repulsive, unacceptable, too kinky. We only have sex in the missionary position in the dark. Regina told me she would NEVER do that and how could I even think that it was okay?" I began to wonder how he reconciled not having the sex he found extremely pleasurable for the last seventeen or so years since marrying his wife.

I imagined this secret was too big and needed more time than this session would allow. I said, "Billy, I know there may be much more you would like to tell me. I am noticing we have about five more minutes of time left, can we pick this up at our next appointment?"

He nodded his head, took a deep breath through his nose, exhaling from his mouth, made direct eye contact with me and he nodded his head, "Yeah Peg, what I want to share is going to need more time. I am so grateful you took the time to asked me sexual questions where my last therapist avoided them like the plague. She and I met for about a year, and I could only start talking about sex after about eleven months of weekly meetings. Once I did start to talk about my sex life, I quickly realized she could not help me. I needed a specialist who dealt with sexual issues. Yes, let's begin with this next session."

The following week I opened the door to the waiting room to see Billy sitting in a chair. I quickly noted his legs were crossed and the top leg was shaking rapidly up and down. He appeared anxious. He stood up swiftly, looked directly into my eyes, and he said, "I am happy to be here." He passed me to enter the meeting space to find a spot on the leather sofa directly under the two side-by-side windows looking out at the light snow falling.

Billy started. "I have to finish what we began discussing last session. I can't hold on to this secret anymore."

"Of course." I said, "please feel free to share."

"I think I must be gay. My girlfriend broke up with me when I was eighteen after I told her I had sex with an older man. My wife has no idea about any of this. I love Regina; our life is so good together, except for our sex life. About seven years ago she stopped wanting sex with me. I started going on gay porn sites, and bought a lot of toys for myself, which I've hidden from her. During that time, I had sex with men I met on the sites. The odd thing is I am not attracted to them. I must be gay, or why else would I go back? How am I ever going to tell her any of this? She is going to flip the fuck out and I just know she'll divorce me. I don't know if I can live without her." He then added, "I can't figure out why I like anal sex, I'm not attracted to men. I just like having sex with them. This filled my craving for anal sex, mainly because men are easily available. I think they wanted it too, maybe for the same reason I did, since most of them were also married."

I nodded my head, remained silent, and I thought about what he was sharing, recalling the book I read by Dr. Joe Kort, *Is My Husband Gay, Straight, or Bi?: A Guide for Women Concerned about Their Men*. And there was another article he had written for *Psychology Today* in August of 2017 titled, "Sexual Disorientation of Male Sexual Abuse Survivors: Sexual abuse disorients you: it doesn't orient you." I also recalled the many different times I consulted with experts in the sex therapy field about this very topic of straight men having sex with men. From my experience, Billy most likely was not gay and reenacting his early childhood experiences through his adult sexual behavior.

I no longer wonder why many of the individuals who find me and want treatment for OCSB—or the many other sexual issues—they find themselves in such precarious situations. From my years studying trauma, I understand how upsetting early childhood events show up in many adults' lives. I was beginning to think this was the case with Billy.

I looked him in the eyes, brought my left palm up to my sternum, took a deep breath, and on the exhale emphatically said, while nodding my head, "Yeah Billy, there is no way to know at this point how she is going to respond." My reaction was automatic and my empathy for Billy brought on these compassionate feelings and my body automatically responded with the action of bringing my hand to my chest. To help him feel at ease I waited a few seconds before I said, "Many couples *do* work through this Billy. There will be a change in the relationship dynamic. It is never going to be the same as before you share this information with her. Many of the couples I see become even more connected. The relationship develops intimacy in a way that they never had before, and they develop a stronger bond. Usually, this requires a lot of therapy for both individuals."

I continued, "In your case, you will need to understand a few things that are going to be entirely new concepts which I will help you to learn. To begin with, how your body's autonomic nervous system is causing you to react in ways that you may not understand, how your emotional system has been trying to protect you for years, and through your eyes it may look like the very behavior you hate that you are doing now. And how to repair yourself to live the life you want to live going forward. In addition, I am pretty sure Regina is going to be heartbroken, angry at you, and upset with herself. Partners of the men I see with OCSB usually are confused; many frequently think they did something wrong to cause you to seek sex outside the marriage. They often have negative thoughts about themselves, which causes them to become insecure and doubt they can ever trust their partner again. Some individuals lash out with fury or rage. One thing I can let you know about: anger is a double-edged sword. One side is anger and the other is vulnerability. The repair of your relationship is going to take time. I have seen many couples pull through this to have even stronger relationships."

This was not going to be the case for Billy. Regina came into the fourth session with him and was very distraught and enraged. Billy talked first and said, "I couldn't hold the secret any longer and I told Regina yesterday."

Regina looked at me directly and without hesitating said, "I am so pissed off at him. He's gay, ruined my life, and we are getting a divorce." I looked over at Billy who was now slumped down, looking at the floor holding his forehead in his hand, and wiping his eyes with a tissue. I could see how distressed he was. Regina continued, "I don't know what he has told you. Do you know he's been having sex with men for many years of our marriage? I could have forgiven him if he was having an affair with another woman. This takes the cake, and I won't have anything to do with this charade of a marriage. I am beyond angry, and I can't ever see myself with him anymore. How can this be? Can you explain any of this to me?"

I began by validating how difficult this must be for her and told her what I thought was happening. I pulled out the book by Dr. Kort, and opened the front cover to pull out the article he had written. I told her what the article was about, but she wouldn't have any of my explanation. She cut me off by saying, "This is bullshit, you don't know what you are doing."

She turned to me—I immediately noticed her body now trembling, her breathing shifted to short hollow breaths, and her eyes darted around the room. She looked back at Billy shouting, "I am DIVORCING HIS SORRY ASS!" She paused and began crying. In an attempt to soothe her Billy reached over to her arm, she turned glaring at him saying, "Don't you touch me. I had an extremely difficult childhood with my fucking parents. You know all about that, you don't see me running around have sex with other people. Especially gay sex. I can't even comprehend what is happening. I am getting a lawyer and ending this."

She stood up and grabbed her red designer handbag and the black and white checkered colored coat she wore into the room. I thought to myself, this isn't black and white like the colors in her coat. The red of her purse reminded me of the foreshadowing in a movie scene where red indicates something bad is about to happen.

Regina briefly looked at me then turned around to Billy and said, "I refuse to hear any more of this ridiculous cover up for your behavior. I am going to my sister's. I am going to stay there. I don't want to see you or hear from you, and I will get my stuff from the house when you aren't there. You're pathetic!" She walked past me, opened the door to the waiting room, walked through it without shutting it, and then opened the door to exit the suite, and slammed it shut.

A few months later Billy and Regina divorced with the help of a mediator. Regina bought a condo and moved into it, while Billy continued his sessions with me. For many more months, I supported Billy. He struggled with depression and huge amounts of grief due to losing Regina. He said, "It feels like she died. I love and miss her so much." In addition, he felt horrible about losing the grandchildren.

Billy and I spent many sessions where he was brokenhearted because he had reached out to Janet, Regina's daughter. She initially promised him she would not let the divorce get in the way of him seeing the kids. Billy tried week after week, texting, emailing, and even talking with Janet a few times. The weeks turned into months and slowly all contact with Janet decreased until it stopped. It was hard to watch Billy. The grandkids' birthdays went by, and a few holidays came and went. Billy was holding onto gifts for his grandchildren. I think he suffered the most from not seeing the youngsters.

Approximately six months into our sessions Billy's loneliness skyrocketed. He had told me he had increased his drinking and wasn't working out physically, which he loved to do. He was depressed and he desperately wanted to understand his sexual orientation. He didn't know if he was gay, straight, bisexual, or even pansexual. He was questioning everything about his identity.

One day I opened the door to the waiting room to see him sitting upright, not slouched in the waiting room chair, and he seemed to spring to his feet. I felt my own body instantaneously: my backbone straightened, and my shoulders relaxed. Our eyes met, and we both smiled. I knew it wasn't because it was a beautiful late summer day, it was something else. He entered the meeting space, and I closed the door. He sat down immediately on the sofa across from me. I looked out the two windows above him; there wasn't a cloud in the sky. I felt the enthusiasm in the air. I looked at him and before I could say a word he spoke, "You are not going to believe what I am going to tell you."

"Try me," I said.

Before he said anything else, I noticed his face. It was flushed with color, his eyes were sparkling, and his smile was ear to ear. I couldn't wait to see what had happened when he was displaying hope for the first time. He began, "you know we have been talking about how I am so confused about my sexual orientation, and you suggested I listen to the podcast on sexual fluidity?

Well, I did take the time to listen to it. I have such relief, and I finally understand it and the name for it, I am heteroflexible!

Now I was smiling ear to ear and asked him, "What does heteroflexible mean to you?"

"Well," he said, "from what I have gathered, I am mainly attracted to women and sometimes I might be drawn to men."

A few weeks later he was struggling with loneliness, and we discussed the possibility of meeting new people or possibly a group of like-minded individuals. He said he had found a site on the web that was very intriguing to him, a social network used by many in the BDSM, fetish, and kink community. He was unsure and wanted my opinion on joining. I encouraged him to go with his gut feelings.

Two weeks later he told me he had joined, and he wanted to tell me all about it. He met a group of people who he felt shared similar interests and they had invited him to an event. Billy wasn't sure what to do. He was nervous and once again asked me what I thought. I asked him about his impressions of the group, and he replied, "I am finding them to be super nice, interesting, and totally open when it comes to talking about sex. I want to go, and they are into swinging. I don't know anything about swinging except what they've told me about. They even said they don't usually let single men join and for some reason they invited me." He looked at me, knew I wouldn't tell him to go or not to go, and asked me my thoughts about swingers.

I smiled, looked at him, then followed by looking out the windows directly above his head. A flock of birds flew by. "Billy" I said, "you know I am going to say to you trust your inner senses." I paused, placed my hand to my chin, and looked down at the ten-inch-high clock shaped like a human being. It sits on the bottom shelf of the coffee table between us, facing me. I saw we had a few more minutes. At last, I looked Billy in the eyes. I said, "swingers, like all people, are multifaceted." I paused, trying to find just the right words to support him in his decision, knowing inside I was jumping for joy. I couldn't exactly share that. I continued, "I think it's important." pausing again, laughing to myself trying not to show it, "that you decide for yourself."

Billy knew my style and began laughing and said, "Do you know the movie with Billy Crystal when he played a psychiatrist and Robert De Niro was his client?"

"Yes," I replied. "Why?"

He continued by imitating De Niro pointing his finger to me, "You, You, you're good..." We both cracked up. Billy understood what I never said in words.

The swinger group accepted Billy without any hesitation, and he began to flourish. He told me how he met ten married couples at the first party he went to. He exclaimed how nice the group was, that they were fun to be around, and how a particular couple whom he felt took him under their wing. The couple had been wedded for over twenty years or longer. Billy was surprised at how much trust they had in one another.

"Regina and I never shared this kind of trust," he said. "It's entirely unlike anything I have ever witnessed in my life. The people are all diverse in every way. It's blown my mind I never knew what to expect— they are totally normal. There are individuals from all walks of life, from a doctor, garage mechanic, to a wealthy businesswoman, accountant, and even a veterinarian!"

I looked at Billy and couldn't hold back my grin and said, "what did you think they were going to be like?"

"I actually didn't know and never expected them to be ordinary people!"

We both laughed out loud. I still smile when I think of that moment, it was precious. I was not taken aback by anything Billy told me. I thought this was going to be what his experience was going to be.

Billy also said, "The couple that I embraced at the party introduced me to 'The Lifestyle,' and I now understand it better. I don't know about any other group, and I really like these people. Many of the couples introduced themselves to me and were so open about how some of the husbands were bi and that's how I fit in so well." He continued, "I had sex with a male/female couple for the first time and discovered I liked the feeling of being fucked by the husband while mentally connecting to his wife. I also found out why they allowed me, a single guy, to join their group. It was because of the type of sex I like! Within the group I can truly be myself without fear of being ridiculed or judged for my sexual desires."

Weeks and months passed, and Billy was still missing Regina, Janet, and the grandchildren. He confided that the group was comforting, but he was still lonely. He told me how "The Lifestyle" group was helping him reinforce the work we were doing in therapy. He started to believe that there was nothing wrong with what he liked, if he was honest with himself, and others, pursued what he liked, and always asked consent from others. His shame was going away.

"Somewhere along the line I stopped worrying about others finding out about my liking anal sex," he said. "I have come to realize that for me to have a great relationship with someone, they have to be willing to please me in that way or it just won't work out in the long run. I began to start meeting women, and if it looks like we might have sex, I will talk to them about what they like and don't like and share what I like and don't like too. I have just started doing this right after we talked about making a list of what I want sexually with anyone or with a future partner. I also think the project where you had me writing about what I saw are my problems, successes, and failures, and how it contributed to the end of feeling and living in shame."

Billy did begin to date. He came in one day again beaming and told me about a woman he met online who was also into swinging. He was very excited about her and perhaps a little too enthused. He admitted she might be the one.

"Billy," I said. "I want to share with you six words that I recently heard, *'Date for fun not the one.'* Does that make any sense to you?" He looked at me a bit confused, so I added, "I wonder if you are going a little too fast here. I know you are still grieving Regina and I don't know if you can find the ONE in the first person you meet online.

He said, "I think I understand what you are saying, but I really like her."

"Okay," I replied. "Just try to take a little more time if you can."

A few weeks went by, and Billy came into his session feeling depressed. He said, "It didn't work out with the woman I met online, she was not the one. She had so much going on she wasn't returning my calls or any of my texts. I have given up on her."

We continued our therapeutic work over the next couple of months until he bounced back and met another woman. "Peg," he said, "this woman is different, and I am not doing the same thing I was with the person I met online. I am taking my time this time. I met her through a mutual friend who has been trying to fix us up. We all met as a group for a drink, her name is Halley, and she isn't what I am usually physically attracted to. There's something about her I am intrigued by."

Another few weeks went by, and Billy was beginning to like Halley a lot, even though she wasn't athletic, or built like Regina, who was trim. Billy said, "I never in my wildest dreams thought I could like someone with a heavier frame, but she's not fat. She's about twenty pounds overweight, and when she goes on hikes with me, she needs to take breaks up the steeper hills, I am okay waiting at the top for her." He also told me how he was going to share everything with Halley as he wanted to start any new relationship that may bloom into a long-term partnership with complete honesty.

Billy did share and told her about his desire for anal sex with his next partner, how the swinging group was now his friends, and how supportive they were. He told her he was in therapy and learned that when he was lonely, he would seek out men for a sexual connection. He admitted that he was scared he would never meet a woman who wouldn't shame him for his yearnings for anal play.

Halley not only understood what he was saying, she replied, "I don't know anything about anal sex, and I have only had sex with a few partners before my ex-husband, and I divorced ten years ago. I would be willing to learn more about it and maybe even try it with you," adding, "I don't know anything about swinging either, but I would also be interested in learning more about it."

Billy told me he was flabbergasted and wondered how this could possibly be that he met someone willing to learn about and possibly try anal play. When he came in one day for his session, he was exuberant. He spoke almost immediately and said, "Peg, you are not going to believe what I am going to tell you."

I replied, "Oh, I think I will, let me hear what you are so enthusiastic about."

He said, "Halley has three kids and one of her daughters has a two-year-old. She introduced me to her daughter and her grandson this past weekend while we were having an afternoon boating trip. Yeah, Halley even owns her own boat. I am not trying to get excited, but I am because she has a grandson!" He then added, "If it works out, I can spoil that little boy as I did my own grandchildren."

Billy shared something else in that session. He spoke about how the last two years of being in therapy were healing for him. "Peg," he said. "I can't believe all the work we have done to date. I no longer feel any shame about my anal play or orientation. You helped me heal from shame—something I thought could never happen. Thank you."

Billy

11

Healing from Grief, Loneliness, and Out of Control Sexual Behavior with Sandplay

Billy, whose story is told in chapter ten of this book, did not begin his therapeutic healing until months into his treatment. He suffered greatly from a broken heart; his wife had declared she never wanted to see him again when she found out that, he was having sex with men. Early in his therapy I learned he had beliefs about himself, "I am not in control," "I am a failure," "I am inadequate," "I can't trust anyone," and many more. I assessed the various treatment techniques I offer and considered what might be helpful. I asked him if he would like to try going into the sandplay room, to work with the miniatures and sand.

"Ahh, no thank you I don't think I am ready to do that," he replied.

"No problem let's do something else," I said.

I asked him if he would be open to using Eye Movement Desensitization Reprocessing (EMDR) which he immediately agreed to do. To begin, I asked him how upsetting each of the beliefs was on a scale of zero to ten, and frequently he would say it was a ten. We worked on each belief until he could say he no longer felt they were upsetting to him, and he could score it as a zero. We continued this practice for approximately seven or eight months. Billy continued to feel shame about his desire for anal sex or some sort of anal stimulation. Although many of these beliefs shifted to a zero, he still felt a deeply rooted shame and loneliness which never ceased. His grief persisted in the loss of Regina, his wife of many years, and he couldn't accept that she really left him. I again asked him if he might like to try working in the sand. This time he readily agreed.

DOI: 10.4324/9781003388302-13

What follows are 14 trays from Billy's series of 30 Kalffian sandplay therapy sessions.

At the time, I only had two rooms in the five-room suite I shared with another therapist. The larger room, approximately 16 feet wide by 18 feet long, was where I sat with clients when not working in the sand. The smaller room, approximately 12 feet square, was my sandplay space. A few hundred miniatures were displayed on the shelving that lined the four walls. In the center of the room, there were two handmade wooden trays, one with dry sand, and the other with wet sand.

The first day Billy entered the room with all the miniatures, he looked around like he never laid eyes on this area of my office before. I watched his gait slowly change; it appeared he was a stranger in a foreign land, and he didn't speak the native tongue. In a way, that would be correct. In this room, the language is not conveyed in verbal form, and it takes shape with metaphors, images, or symbols. This is the psyche's vernacular. I made a point of behaving differently in this room, indicating a distinction between the two forms of sand therapy. In the other room—designed to make the clients feel more at home in a living room-like setting—we would rely on talk therapy, freely discussing issues, and using our common language.

I am sure Billy noticed the shift in my presence, too, I became much less talkative. My major role as a Kalffian sandplay practitioner is to become an attuned silent witness for clients, allowing them to trust their own instincts. Billy's psyche was going to direct him on how to heal from all the shame he was carrying for his desire to engage in anal stimulation in his sexual play. I didn't know how many trays he would make in his Kalffian sandplay series; I knew this therapy would shift his core beliefs and shame.

"Billy, I told you at our last meeting, this is going to be a different type of session. While we are in this room, you are going to work in the sand and complete a sandplay tray. I am not going to give you any guidance on what miniatures to pick. I am just going to sit where I will be out of the way so you can take as much time as you need to look at all the miniatures on the shelves. There isn't any right or wrong way to do this, just choose what comes to you."

"Okay, I will give it a shot, I don't have any idea where to even start." he said. He moved around the room surveying his options.

Beginning on the left of the room, he walked around the space and carefully selected a few miniatures. Once he finished, he stood in front of the tray with dry sand and placed the following items: a white mountain, a Wonder Woman figure, a fireman holding a baby, a T. Rex dinosaur, a boat, and a white faceless female yoga figure. Then he sat down to look at what his tray looked like. I moved to the chair on his right-side and sat next to him. See Figure 11.1.

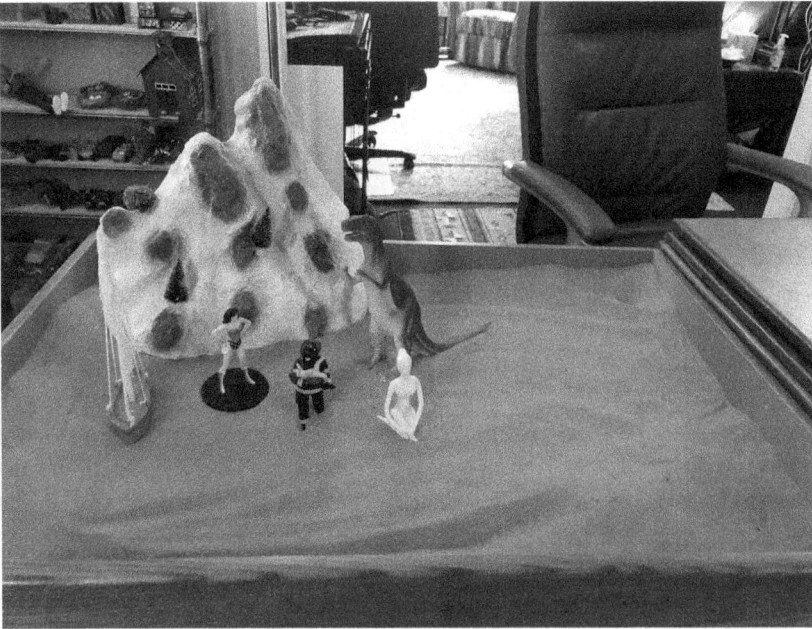

Figure 11.1 The Mountain with Dinosaur and Other Miniatures

Photo by the author

I waited for him to look at me after he placed all the miniatures in the tray. "Billy, does this *feel* complete?" I asked.

"Yeah, I guess so," he said.

"Okay, would you like to share anything about this world?"

"The dinosaur is my grandson, Wonder Woman is my Regina, the sailboat represents how much I love to sail. I don't know why I chose the mountain, yoga figure, or the fireman with the baby." He paused and I waited, nodding my head to reassure him I was completely present. He looked at me and then back at the scene in the tray.

"Billy, where's the energy in the tray?" I asked.

"The energy in the tray is the mountain, it's just peaceful, and natural, I guess. It's white so it's clear and pure. The white yoga figure is sexuality. It's someone who is confident, natural, and secure." He paused again. I waited silently for him to continue at his pace, and I wondered if that female yoga figure was also his vision of what he thought his partner should look like, a slim-waisted female with big breasts, like his ex-wife Regina. Bill, in Chapter 10 had shared in a session how he was attracted only to slim women and how they turned him on. He said he wasn't attracted to anyone with a heavier frame and especially not women he considered to be overweight. I pondered if this yoga figure would change during his sandplay process. What was Billy's psyche saying to him without using words? I knew in sandplay the psyche often utilizes symbols that may change form during the process, the person's perspective can change externally.

Approximately two minutes later he spoke again. "I love to help people with their problems," he said. "I especially love helping kids and I have a big thing if anyone hurts kids. And oh, I see I forgot the fireman holding the baby. That's how I help people." He gazed at the scene again, adding, "I love the yoga figure it's so calm."

In a matter of a few seconds Billy got up from his chair, walked over to the shelves, and grabbed a second mountain. I had asked an artisan to custom-make this piece around the time I was working with a mountain in my own process. I designed it with a very shear façade on one side. On the other side was an easier side, with a path, waterfall, and a hairpin turn. Billy placed the steep vertical side facing us on the right side of the tray which he had left empty (Figure 11.2).

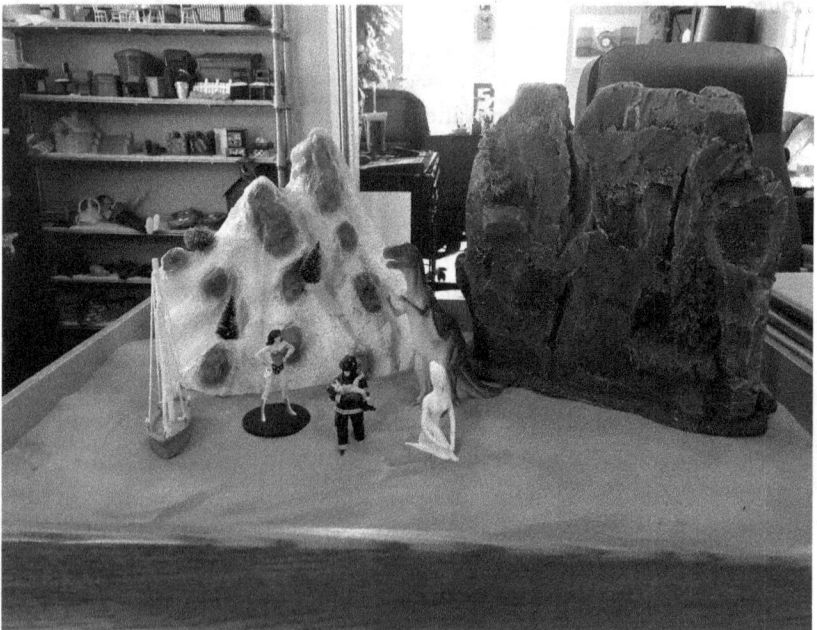

Figure 11.2 Two Mountains

Photo by the author

"I actually feel like the white mountain is too easy to get over," he said. "This gray mountain is harder, and it's meant for me. Nobody can climb that mountain. Nobody."

We sat in silence for approximately four minutes until he spoke again, only this time, his voice was cracking, and tears were welling up in his eyes. He reached over to the grey mountain, held it in the air, and placed it directly in front of himself. The top of the mountain was just above his eyes. He couldn't see any of the other miniatures behind it either. It was a powerful moment when he articulated the only words he could.

"This is how I feel," he whispered.

He hung his head down into his hands. His entire face was hidden until he looked up and wiped away his tears. I knew that he was feeling shame (Figure 11.3).

During the next few sessions Billy discussed how he had met a new group of individuals on an adult website, this was the same group he mentioned in chapter ten. He was surprised to find they had very open attitudes about sex, were non-judgmental, and were swingers. He was exuberant when he spoke about them and was surprised to hear some of the men were

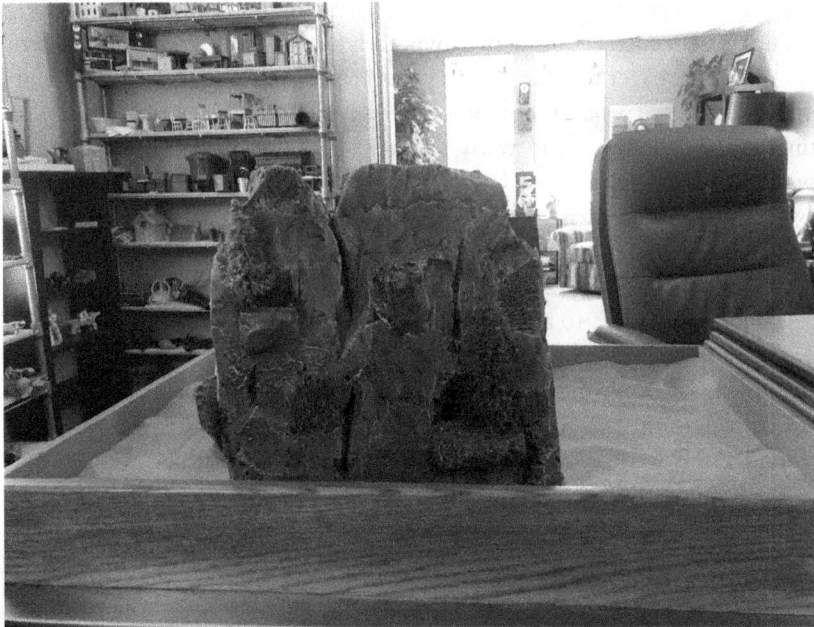

Figure 11.3 This Is How I Feel

Photo by the author

partnered or married to women, shared that they were bi-sexual, and would love to meet him. Billy was extremely curious about what it would be like to meet up with them, and he ultimately decided to accept an invitation to one of their parties. After meeting with them at the party, he told me how much he enjoyed their company; couldn't believe the variety of the people he was meeting. "I can't believe it," he said. "They are all normal folks."

I smiled when he used the word, "normal" to describe the individuals in the group.

"What kind of person did you expect?" I asked.

"I actually wasn't sure what to expect, they are great individuals."

During these sessions Billy and I continued discussing his growing fondness, trust, and friendships with this group of swingers. During this sandplay session is when he told me he recently went to a party with the group and had sex with a married couple. In addition, he added how he realized he preferred sex with the woman, not the man, and how he felt genuine with her.

A few weeks later Billy had the divorce meeting with the mediator and his soon to be ex wife. This occurred earlier in the morning, prior to his therapy appointment with me. When I opened the door to the waiting room, he was smiling ear to ear, quickly got up from his seat, and said, "I can't wait to share what happened at the mediation meeting this morning!" I found myself smiling and recognized how my own body was reacting to his enthusiastic energy. I was eager to hear what he was about to tell me. I walked into my office, closed the waiting room door, and sat in my chair. He was already sitting on the sofa, leaning forward on the edge of the cushion. I could see he was energized.

"I am so proud of myself," he said. "I am beginning to understand my sexual desire for anal play doesn't mean I am gay or sick. I was able to say this today to Regina for the first time at our mediation meeting this morning."

I understood how, to a self-identified heterosexual male, labels such labels gay or bi might exacerbate feelings of shame and insecurity. I reminded him that there was no shame in desiring anal intercourse, nor in admitting homosexual feelings. I assured him that he didn't need to label his behavior, and should, instead, consider why this brought on such shame.

He waited a moment. "I want to share with you what I said to Regina. Are you ready?"

"Of course, I can't wait for you to share," I said. "You are beaming from the inside out."

"I said this to Regina: 'You left me, and I now know I am not gay or bisexual. The only thing I am guilty of is I like anal stimulation and that's not anything to be ashamed of." In my practice, I treat a wide range of clients, all who self-identify with a diversity of sexual orientations and gender identities. I am careful not to assign my own labels to my clients, allowing them the freedom to express themselves.

I was impressed he could now recognize his sexual pleasure wasn't odd or disgusting, but rather a natural expression of his desires. When he ceased to think of himself in terms of labels that may or may not have negative connotations in his mind, he was free to explore his own wants and needs. Through the Kalffian sandplay modality, Billy had accessed a deeper aspect of himself, where words didn't confer negative connotations. I wondered just how much of his shame had lifted.

Within moments he asked me if he could make a sandplay tray. I was very curious about what this tray would look like and told him of course he could do a tray. This time he selected seven miniatures: the white mountain, a rock with the word sister on it, another rock engraved with the word trust, a small pyramid, a small white figure holding its head in its hands, a teal figure without any facial features, and a bridge. I was thrilled to see he picked a bridge. The bridge can represent—among many things—an attempt to connect one thing to another. Yet, the placement of this bridge displayed something unknown in an empty area closest to where he was sitting nearest to the mountain. Time would tell what was trying to connect with or to. I asked Billy if he wanted to share anything about this world. "The usual mountain is back. I think that is where I am going. It's a trust thing and I want to have people trust me." When he said that, I thought about how he was building trust with the swingers.

"I have no idea of the teal guy with his legs crossed is all about, but it's at peace."

I thought about what he said to Regina and how he was more comfortable and seemed more at peace with himself.

"The white one is what's going on tonight. The swingers are coming over to my house." he said.

I looked at the white non-binary figure that had its head down, butt up in the air, and thought about how Billy enjoyed the anal play. This white figure was located directly behind the teal figurine he said was peaceful. Maybe he wasn't completely at peace; this white figure could also have represented his sadness about the divorce and missing the children (Figure 11.4).

He added, "I recently had a guy come over to have sex and I told him I wasn't into it. I just didn't want to do it with him once he got to my place. It didn't feel right." He paused again. "The couple and the swingers have been so nice to me. I invited them over for sex tonight. I am going to join them because I like them, trust them, and they helped me out by supporting me."

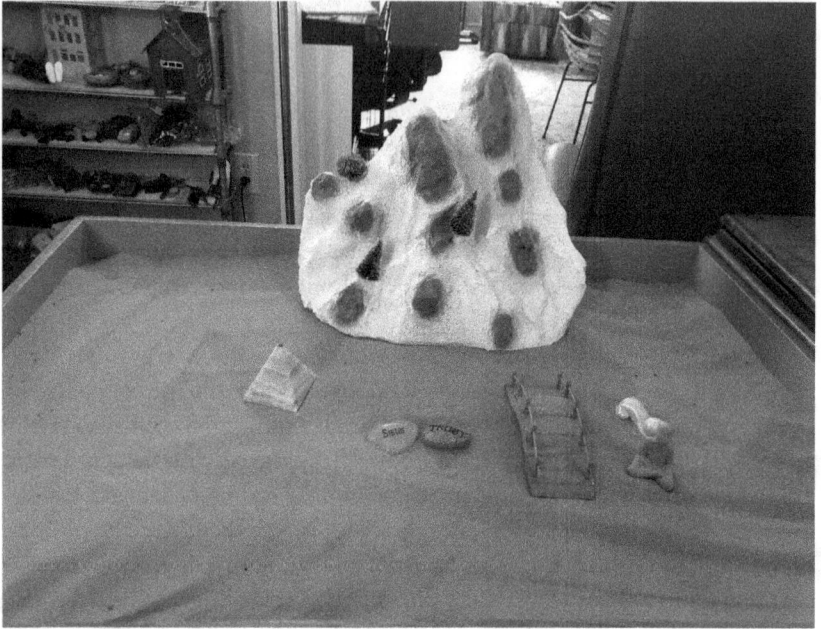

Figure 11.4 Trust Tray

Photo by the author

After he completed the tray, he shared the following "I am thinking about the last swinging party. I didn't put the other mountain in because I didn't need it. I'm over that hurdle and on my way to a fresh start."

He looked at the tray again, his smile slipping a bit. "Once my ex-wife gets all her money. I'm worried it will be all over with my connection with the grandchildren. I will miss those kids. At their last soccer game, they asked if I would go over to their house, I didn't know what to do." He had tears in his eyes when he talked about losing the grandchildren.

At that moment he recalled an episode about the teenage boys taking advantage of him in the woods. The sudden outpouring of emotion surrounding the loss of his grandchildren opened an emotional connection to that traumatic childhood experience. The two were linked in his system. This was the first time he told me about his trauma story. Yet he didn't even realize he wasn't talking *to me*; he was talking aloud *to himself*. I was acutely aware of his need for my complete presence, so I ceased taking notes. I don't have verbatim quotations and I remembered the first sentence. "I was only four years old, that's not shown here in this tray," he mumbled.

In sandplay the trauma story evolves naturally. By waiting for the story to arise in its own pace, Billy was able to share his trauma story and tolerate the emotions which arose. Lorraine Freedle, in her 2017 article "Healing trauma through sandplay therapy: A neuropsychological perspective," discusses the four components of sandplay that are interrelated in healing trauma from a neuropsychological point of view. She writes, "Sandplay therapy is relational, experiential, and sacred. From a neuropsychological perspective, four interrelated mechanisms of Sandplay therapy drive the therapeutic process. These have relevance for people who have experienced trauma. Together these aspects of Sandplay promote neural integration" (pp. 190–205). The four mechanisms are listed below:

1. relational safety and "generous attunement"
2. somatosensory engagement
3. symbolic expression of the trauma narrative
4. mindful participation

Freedle further discusses in the article how multiple brain systems are activated during neural integration while working in the sand in the effective treatment of trauma. She writes, "Four interrelated mechanisms of Sandplay therapy promote neural integration with particular relevance for people who have experienced trauma: relational safety and generous attunement by the therapist open neural pathways for social engagement and implicit mutual influence; somatosensory engagement provides a way to access and reprocesses trauma through the body and the sensory system; symbolic expression of the trauma narrative stimulates connections within and between brain regions, develops internal resources, and expands conscious awareness; and, last, mindful participation enhances self-regulatory capacities and higher order consciousness" (pp. 190–205).

Kalff in her book, *Sandplay: A Psychotherapeutic Approach to the Psyche*, the color addition, writes, "Therefore, I have taken it as my task in therapy to create a free and protected space for the child within our relationship. The free space comes into being in the therapeutic setting when the therapist can fully accept the child and is able to participate internally just as intensely as does the child in everything that happens. When the child senses that he or she is not alone in distress or happiness, the child feels free and protected to express whatever is moving within" (p. 5).

By holding space for Billy, I gave him the freedom to share with me his childhood ordeal for the first time.

Deb Dana in her book, *The polyvagal Theory in Therapy: Engaging in the Rhythm of Regulation* calls this co-regulation and writes, "Through co-regulation, a foundation of safety is created, and attachment follows. Co-regulation creates a physiological platform of safety that supports a psychological story of security that then leads to social engagement" (p. 44).

It is when two autonomic nervous systems connect when individuals feel safe. It is in these moments of safety clients can share many upsetting events with an attuned therapist. This sandplay tray was a breakthrough for Billy, connecting him with traumatic events he had, most likely, not processed or even mentioned aloud, even to himself.

To describe this further Kay Bradway, a Jungian analyst and founding member of the C.G. Jung Institute coined the term *co-transference*. In Bradway's article, "Transference and countertransference in sandplay therapy," she writes, "I preferred the term co-transference which indicates a feeling *with*, rather than a feeling of *against*. Currently I tend to use the term co-transference to designate the therapeutic feeling relationship. These inter-feelings seem to take place more simultaneously than the composite term transference / countertransference suggests" (p. 29). I believe Billy's ability to communicate his trauma was a combination of 'the free and protected space' inter-feelings we shared, and the connection of our autonomic nervous systems.

Billy continued to share more about his tray. "The teal miniature is at peace now. It's a man, not the yoga figure I used in that first tray." I wondered if he was the teal man at peace now that he told me his trauma story. Did the psyche know he was going to share all that he shared while he was picking the miniatures that session?

One-week later Billy came into my office. When I opened the door, I noticed he was not happy, like he was on his last visit. He appeared visibly upset. When he entered the room he said to me, "I am feeling collapsed in my personal life and unable to perform at my job."

"Billy what's going on?" I asked. We both sat down.

He collapsed onto the sofa. "I almost went on a double date. I experienced fear when I thought about talking with someone about my past sexual experiences. I'm thinking about contacting men for sex."

"Is there more about that?" I asked.

He continued, "I have been crying a lot and feel horrible about myself. I don't know. I just don't have any vision and I haven't gone back to work yet. The first quarter of my work is screwed, I just don't want to do it even though I know I must. I don't want to go on a vacation alone and I don't want to go with friends. I miss Regina, I'm lonely. I'm forcing myself to fit in having sex, and I am not enjoying it."

Nodding my head, looking at him, I placed my hand over my heart, took a deep breath, and I found myself emitting a sound before I spoke. "Hmmm."

I felt it vibrate in my throat. "Billy," I said, then paused. "I know how much Regina meant to you." I let him sit with that. Finally, I said, "Would you like to work in the sand today?"

He nodded his head. We entered the sandplay room and he slowly moved around. I sat in a chair nearby. He selected six figures: a much smaller mountain, a bridge with snow on it, a small non-binary gray figure lying down—which, he placed halfway under the bridge, a coral scene, the teal figure from the last tray, now placed on its side, a scuba diver, and a shark positioned directly under the scuba diver (Figure 11.5).

When asked about this world he said, "I am thinking I am going to need to take a trip just to get away. I want to scuba dive or some other kind of trip, maybe a cruise ship, and I don't typically do cruises. I have no idea what the two figures mean. The bridge is getting me to where I am going. I don't have any vision of where that is and that's why I put the little mountain in the back. The energy in the tray is the scuba diver." He paused and added, "I'm just hiding. That's why I put the bridge on top of the gray figure. That's me, I'm not happy with myself." He paused for about one and a half minutes.

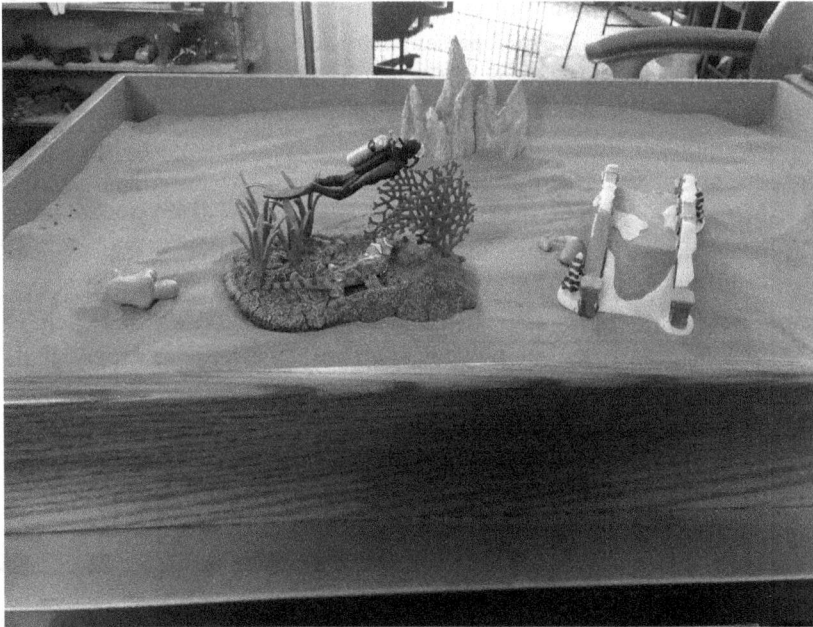

Figure 11.5 The Scuba Diver

Photo by the author

I thought about this tray and the symbolism in it. I contemplated how the mountain had changed dramatically. It was smaller, with peaks and valleys, possibly representing what life was like for Billy now, moments of summits where he would feel joyfulness—like he had last week when he had clarity and spoke his truth to Regina—then other periods of melancholy and isolation. When people feel isolated, the autonomic nervous system moves into a survival response, and it doesn't feel safe. This is a physiological human condition and happens naturally when individuals will reach out to feel some type of connection with another person. This explained to me Billy's periodic reaching out to men for sex and how he was having sex with members of the group and not necessarily enjoying it at this time.

The scuba diver may have been a symbol representing Billy's observing ego witnessing his collapsed and vulnerable state shown by the gray figure on its side, embodying Billy's distressing emotional state. The diver was looking directly at the curled-up gray figure Billy identified as himself, placed halfway under the partially snow-covered bridge; it appeared to bear witness to his pain. This bridge had elements of the cold mountain in the last tray, yet it was unknown if the snow was melting or thawing, so it could conceivably represent an element of hope.

The two human figures in the tray were on their sides, lying down. All symbols in a sandplay tray represent the sand player. I wondered about the teal figure on the left side of the scuba diver. In his previous tray, he said the teal figure was at peace yet in this tray the teal figure is prone, lying motionless, does not appear to be peaceful, and seems to be in a distressed state. This felt to me emblematic of Billy's own emotional discomfort further amplified by the second gray figure on its side halfway under the bridge. In sandplay when an image duplicates like this, the psyche may be displaying something that is exceedingly important to the sand player, something that has yet to be worked through. In Billy's case, I believe this was his shame and or possibly the depression he was experiencing at that time.

Often, after a huge breakthrough session (for instance, Billy's last tray—where he was able to tell Regina he was not feeling guilty about his wanting anal play—was revelatory), the next sandplay tray may swing naturally in the opposite direction, with an equal and opposite influence. In this tray, Billy seems to be rebounding into a sense of despair which may have been an indication of him beginning to work on his shadow. In Jungian terms, the shadow is what human beings don't like to see in themselves and must face to transform. This is a way the psyche expands towards healing by facing shadow on multiple planes, first on a personal level, then on a collective one. The individual must face and feel their own internal pain—or shame in the case of Billy—on a deeper archetypal level, the shadow of the world's pain or shame.

With each subsequent tray, the work goes deeper, having to first go into the light before plunging into the dark. We call this "higher in order to go deeper" to reach the level of the soul. In Billy's tray, the diver may be looking or exploring for the soul. Donald Kalsched, a Jungian analyst writes in his book, *Trauma and the Soul: A Psycho-Spiritual Approach to Human Development and Its Interruption*, "When the personality is forced to dis-integrate in this way, it is hard on the soul. The soul cannot thrive and grow in the fragmented personality. Its preferred medium is the psycho-somatic integrate, with all the capacities of the self-represented as parts of a whole" (p. 20).

I thought about Freedle's neuropsychological perspective of neural integration, discussed above, the second mechanism of somatosensory engagement, and how sandplay contributes to psychic wholeness by using the sand and miniatures when working with an attuned therapist. Kalsched continues, "This is because the soul *is* by definition, this very animation and aliveness— the center of our God-given spirit—the vital spark in us that 'wants' to incarnate in the empirical personality but needs help from supportive persons in the environment to do so-help that is often not available" (p. 20). In sandplay, the affirmative relationship between the therapist and client is considered a crucial element in healing.

In his next sandplay, Billy selected eight miniatures: the scuba diver, a coral reef with a sand shark underneath, a cheerleader, money, the white yoga figure from the first tray, a wooden bridge, a small clock, and Charlie Brown (Figure 11.6). After making the tray Billy immediately smiled at me and said, "No mountain! I don't know where I am going, maybe I've been creating a mountain out of a molehill."

When I asked him about the world he created, he said, "the bridge is still going somewhere." I noticed one end of the bridge was directly in front of the place where he was now sitting, the other end aimed towards the coral reef area was possibly significant as well. Billy was going deeper into his unconscious. The scuba diver was no longer floating on the top of the reef rather hidden behind the green grass and red coral, at an awkward angle. The scuba diver may have been looking at the cheerleader, but its view was obstructed by the red coral. The diver may have indicated Billy hitting rock bottom placed on the base of the coral miniature. Then he said, "the cheerleader could cost me a lot of money. I don't have a budget for that." I saw the money next to the cheerleader and wondered if he feared being in another relationship due to the financial situation of his pending divorce. The money in the tray could also symbolize Billy's sense of self-worth and value.

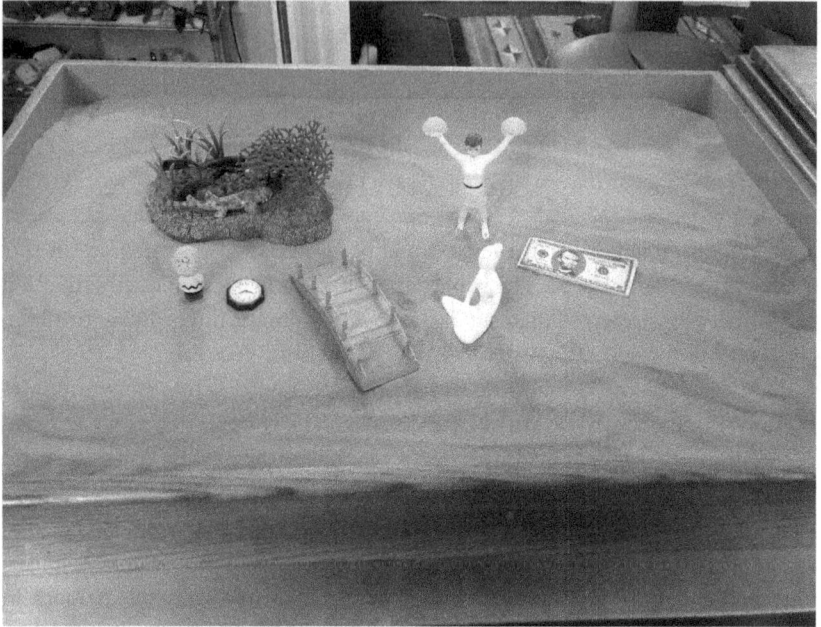

Figure 11.6 The Bridge to Somewhere

Photo by the author

He added, "last night I dreamed of me and my dad in a casino. My dad took his key, money, and he had chips. I think I need to start dreaming of moving on in life." The currency may have been reflective of his dad, or his fear about Regina draining his funds. He continued, "I have to do stuff before I run out of time, and I don't want to be an idiot like Charlie Brown. That yoga figure is me trying to be calm." I noticed the clock next to Charlie Brown on the left side of the bridge. Billy's words felt forced, and I thought he was feeling some sort of self-induced pressure. Maybe the clock was his unconscious showing his conscious mind it was time to do the deeper work.

He closed the session by looking at the center of the tray, adding, "The scuba diver is me on vacation. I want to go away for a week and do it on my own. I will pick something. Maybe, Club Med. I know I'm going to meet someone, and that gives me incentive to work out. Could be new energy entering my system." When I heard him discuss new energy I smiled, and we ended the session.

Billy continued his sandplay therapy, still missed Regina, and wanted to date someone, yet was having difficulties with continued feelings of shame. We had a couple of sessions without using the sand, just talking. For our next session, he wanted to do another sandplay tray, and he briefly told me about how he spent the past weekend and how blissful it was. He said he stayed over at the home of the couple he trusted the most. They were having a weekend party. Billy spoke about how much he enjoyed the get-together, men, and women touching him, and how he slept all night with a single woman who was new to the group. He was proud when he told me he had brought her coffee in the morning—something he would always do for Regina. He found great pleasure in that small gesture.

Billy entered the sandplay room and collected three miniatures: a bridge, a couple with the taller figure in the back, supporting a woman, its arms wrapped around her waist, and a small white non-binary figure. He said, "I don't feel I'm going over any water, so I picked a low bridge. It's not a big bridge, it's a smaller one. I feel like I am closing in. It's an easier bridge to cross." He paused for about two minutes before adding, "the bridge is to find love." At this moment he began to cry.

"I guess I don't feel I have a lot of love, I don't have someone close to be with, and I haven't had that for a fucking long time. Even with my wife…after seven years when everything started changing. I felt closer to that girl I slept with over the weekend. The couple standing in the tray has to be me and the girl I slept with," he said when he pointed to the couple in the tray. I remained quiet, nodding my head; he looked me in the eyes.

"Seven years into my marriage with Regina is when I started playing with guys. What the hell is it about seven years? It's time for my own experiences and it's time to cross that bridge" he said, then pausing for several minutes. "I am looking at the white figure lying down. That's me trying all new sexual stuff I never tried before. I am now experimenting with all things I wanted to try and never did. I got flogged at the party and I liked it," he declared (Figure 11.7).

Before making his next sandplay tray, Billy shared all was going well. He was still drinking and finding it hard to stop. He said he was lonely, missing Regina, and grieving her leaving him. Dr. Jeffrey Rediger writes about loneliness in his book *Cured: The Life-Changing Science of Spontaneous Healing*, "… when we lose the ability to connect, our lizard brains kick in, and we regress to more primitive forms of coping" (p. 193). With the loss of connection Billy's coping mechanism became his drinking—a way to numb out his feelings and not feel his emotional pain from losing his wife. Louis Cozolino, an American psychologist, in his book, *The Neuroscience of Human Relationships: Attachment and The Developing Social Brain* writes, "The psychological and physical symptoms of grief in people who lose a spouse can continue for 5 or more years" (pp. 249–250). Cozolino adds, "While a regular

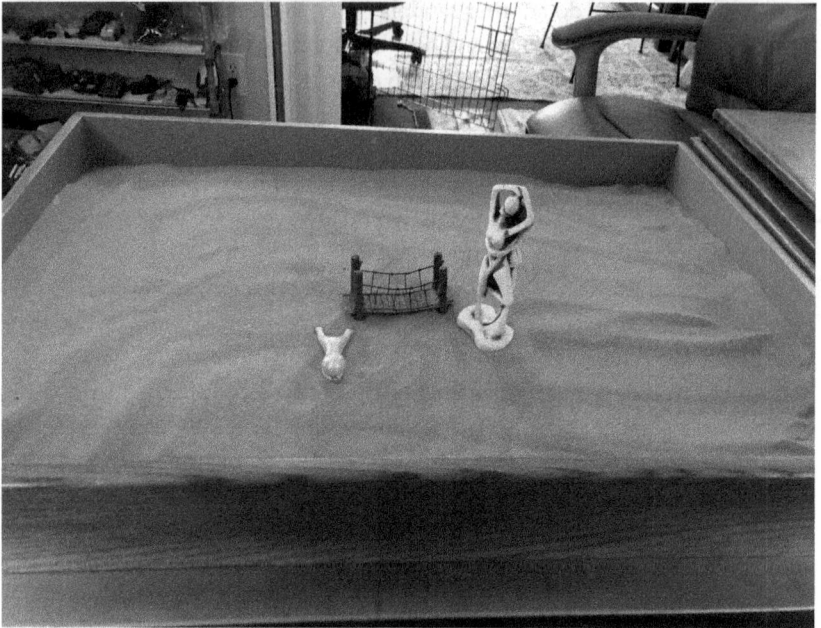

Figure 11.7 The Low Bridge

Photo by the author

dose of voluntary solitude can make an important contribution to emotional balance and self-awareness, imposed isolation can be painful, debilitating, and even worse. Isolation, loneliness, and depression have been shown to have synergistic effect in diminishing well-being that results in reduced autonomic regulation ..." (pp. 249–250).

This is in alignment with Dr. Stephen Porges' Polyvagal Theory. In a personal correspondence on October 3rd, 2021, Porges stated, "The Polyvagal Theory would deconstruct grief, loss, or loneliness as a disruptor of our biological mandate to connect. Without the other to co-regulate with our social engagement systems may become inaccessible and we might seek out external means to regulate our physiology. These strategies may be viewed as addictions or asocial. To the nervous system the strategies are valiant attempts to regulate physiological state to move out of shutdown states."

In Porges' article, "Polyvagal theory: A Biobehavioral Journey to Sociality," he wrote, "The theory emphasizes the need for social interactions in regulating the human autonomic nervous system and in fostering homeostatic functions" (p. 10069). In other words, human beings require connection with others to function both emotionally and physiologically at their best, nurturing stability for optimal survival. Billy found this type of connection with the girl he slept overnight with, and he found himself wanting to bring her coffee in the morning. A very social and regulated thing to do.

In Billy's next sandplay session he entered the sandplay room and walked slowly around the space looking at all the miniatures on the shelves. He spent approximately 15 minutes in silence going to each section, looked from the top to the bottom, and finally he stopped at the non-binary figurines. These figures were custom designed for me by an artisan whom I asked to make them without the physical traits of male or female, shape them in human form, and have each one formed in the shape of an emotion. For example, I have one that is a body curled up in the fetal position, which is used frequently when individuals feel rejected, depressed, or even suicidal.

Billy selected one figure that had its arms crossed, lowered head, and one leg placed under the other. This figure had a headband of rainbow-colored beads. Billy held the miniature for a few seconds, looked at me, shrugged his shoulders, and said, "This is the only one that fits for me today." He then placed it in the center of the tray (Figure 11.8).

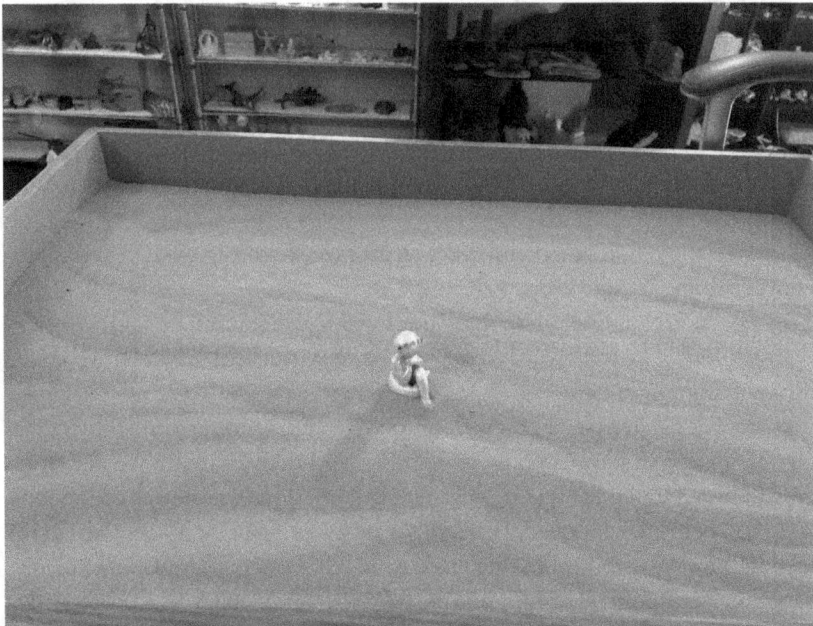

Figure 11.8 Billy's Jeweled Miniature

Photo by the author

When asked about the tray, Billy stated, "this is kind of how I feel, so alone. Alone and I feel it in my body and in my chest. There are empty sensations, nothing there. I have lost everything important to me." He paused for about two minutes and added, "I am killing myself with the thoughts of the first woman I had sex with who broke up with me when I was eighteen. And yesterday I was sitting at a light while driving and I wanted to drive into a pole."

I thought about his last sandplay of connection and now he was having the opposing state of disconnection and loneliness. He was dealing with his reality of living by himself, now having to deal with the sadness, and becoming an emotional being. He shared his feelings of isolation, being alone, craving companionship, and how he loved Regina, and the girl he recently slept with. All this came up when he *thought* about the girl who wouldn't have sex with him when he was in his youth. Only this time he wasn't distracting himself with sex or drugs. He was feeling the distress and tolerating it. I wondered if he was going to start to ascend, starting a new chapter in his life. The little white figure-bejeweled with a rainbow of gems gave me a glimmer of hope.

I asked Billy if he was suicidal and he said, "No way. I know I am grieving Regina and upset about the girl I dated when I was eighteen, and no one is worth killing myself over. That moment at the stop light was fleeting. I know I have to get myself together and get back to thinking about my work."

I nodded and asked, "Billy, I have an idea and wondering if you might be okay if I gave you a homework assignment for our next meeting. Would you be willing to try it?"

"Absolutely it's a big yes from me. What is it you want for me to do?" he asked.

"I would love it if you could make an art piece showing what you want for your life going forward."

"Peg, I don't know how to draw but I will figure it out," he said.

"Fabulous. I look forward to seeing you next week," I said, and we ended our meeting.

Two weeks later I opened my door to the waiting room to find Billy radiating; he appeared stimulated by something, and then I saw the poster board next to him. I looked at it and I completely got it. His energy was contagious, and I too became energized. I couldn't wait to see what he made. During the session, he spoke about how he enjoyed making the collage. Janet, Regina's daughter, had contacted him and he saw the grandchildren in person. He enthusiastically said, "You're not going to believe this. I loved doing the collage so much I purchased age-appropriate magazines for the kids, art materials, and we all made collages. We had so much fun! Then I went to my monthly meeting with my peers. I had called them, told them I wanted to change the meeting a little bit, asked them all to bring art supplies to the meeting, and they did. Peg, I told them what you sometimes say to me when I do a sandplay tray, 'don't think, just pick what comes to you.' They LOVED the project. I couldn't believe it."

"I am so happy for you," I said.

He then discussed how he didn't drink before he hooked up with a gay man. He was not feeling guilty or shameful after he had sex with him, and he was feeling so much more relief in his body (Figure 11.9).

In his next session he did something he never did before. He chose to work in the tray that had wet sand—although he never physically touched the sand. When asked about his tray he said, "I don't know. I am thinking about what I want to do for vacation. Something with water and not a cruise ship. Maybe with a sailboat. I am not sure." He paused. "Why I picked the white figures, I don't know. I think I want companionship. Yeah, I hooked up with a guy over the weekend. I was honest with him, and I told him I was in a swinger group. I am not going to hide that from anyone now. I didn't use my real name or mention that I owned my own business. I know his real name. He's older

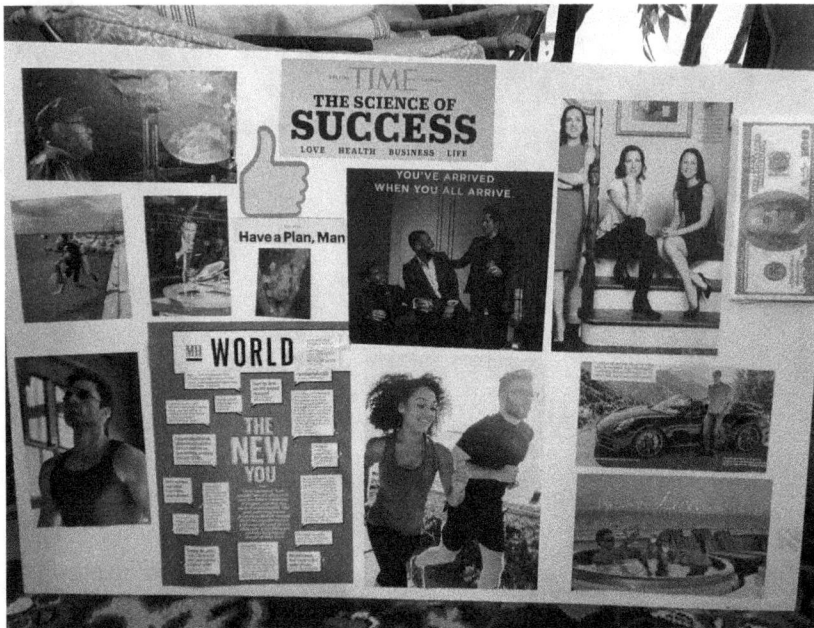

Figure 11.9 Success Board

Photo by the author

than me, in his mid-sixties. It's interesting how it's such a small world. He knows people I know. I told him I'm heteroflexible and attracted to women. I am looking more for a female partner now and I am seeking out people who are into fetish."

I looked at the tray and I had a sense that Billy was healing. I noticed the sand looked like waves on the ocean, a rough sea, and how at peace the white figures looked holding hands. I saw the scuba diver in the tray, he was not on the base but rather floating, looking directly at the white figures. I was pleased to see how the scuba diver had ascended from the rock bottom in the earlier tray to a more balanced state in this one. While underwater, a diver reaches neutral buoyancy—they are not too heavy or too light, and their body is calm. I loved it when I saw how both the diver and the miniature shark were looking at the white figures, especially after Billy commented he didn't know why he picked them. That's the beauty of sandplay, where the unconscious will bring to consciousness to the sandplayer. This often fore-shadows what is going to happen later (Figure 11.10).

Billy's next sandplay session was surprising. He used some figures he had passed over many times before. Prior to placing any miniatures in the tray, he

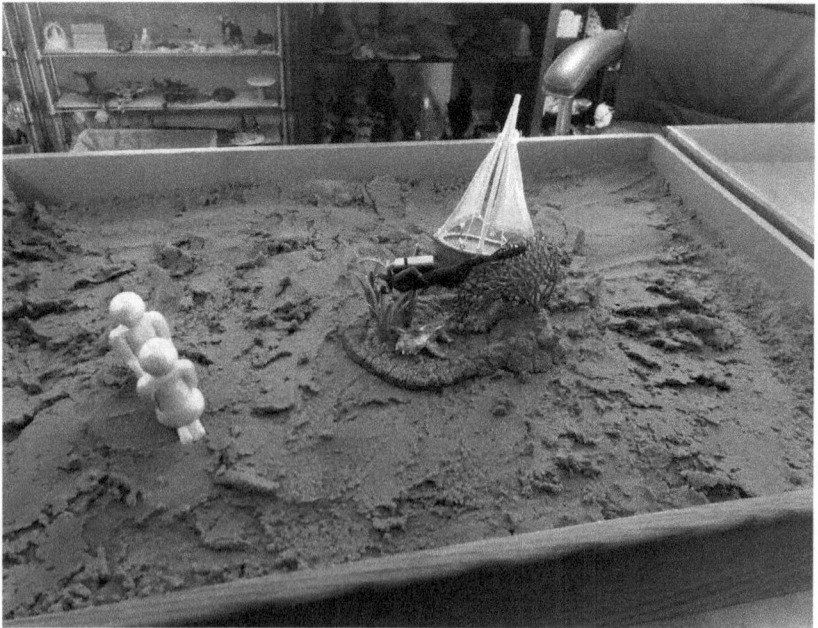

Figure 11.10 The Connected Couple

Photo by the author

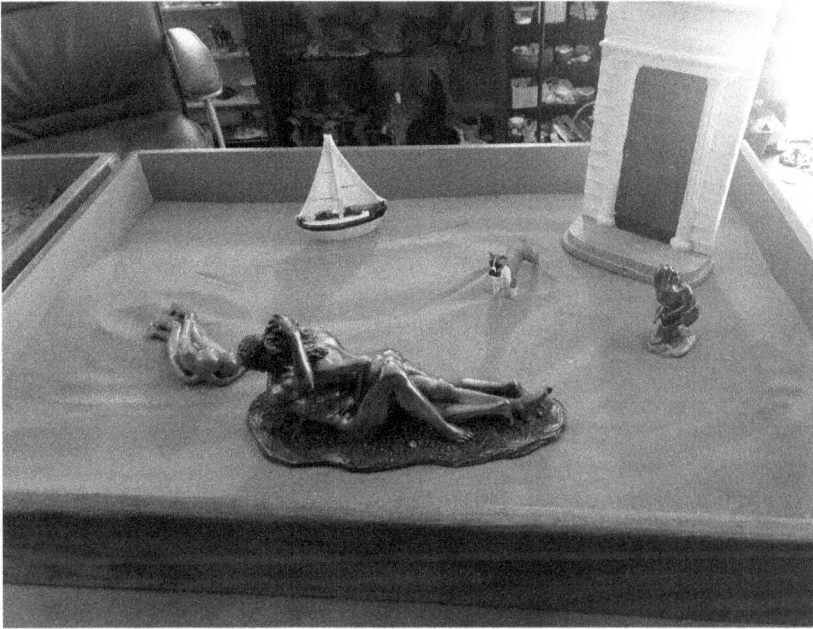

Figure 11.11 Two Couples

Photo by the author

shyly said, "I pulled stuff off the sex shelf. I have always avoided that shelf. I walked past it, and I knew I had to go back. It's time I look at all the sexual parts of me, and I didn't want to pull the ones of the naked women who were alone. So, I picked the nude couple." I watched him place six miniatures into the tray: a large, bronzed couple, a smaller rainbow-colored non-binary couple, a multi-colored Kokopelli, a dog, a large door, and a sailboat (Figure 11.11).

When asked about his world he stated, "The sailboat is me going on a trip on the water." I was amazed at how his last tray felt ocean-like to me, and now he was talking about going on a trip on the water. Often in sandplay, sand players will expose the blue base to represent the ocean or some type of water, Billy didn't do that, yet he was on his journey, and gave himself a vehicle, a sailboat, to take him wherever he was going. The ocean often represents the depths of the unconscious of the psyche.

He continued, "The doorway is not feeling comfortable in my own house because of thoughts of Regina." I wondered about what messages his unconscious was trying to convey to him with this closed red door framed with columns. Maybe he was not yet open to having a partner enter his home space. He continued, "The dog is a loyal companion." I noticed he talked about loyalty and how important that was to him. The dog signified a very safe living mammal, one he could trust, devoted, reliable, and a dedicated fellow traveler on this voyage. Dogs also can be guards to protect us. I noticed it was standing in front of the door on the left side, and it occurred to me that the breed of dog was a boxer. I wondered if the word "boxer" was a metaphor for the unconscious, and Billy was ready to fight for his own survival.

He said, "the Kokopelli is Native American, and it focuses on music, and I love music. The big bronze figure ..." he paused for a few moments, "I want to be with a woman and have a sexual relationship whereas the multi-colored couple figure means intimacy to me."

I thought about both of the couple of miniatures he placed on top of the sand. The first bronze one was the most realistic symbol of the human connection he had picked so far in his sandplay trays. The non-binary couple he picked was featureless. He pointed to this multi-colored couple and welled up with tears.

"I'm not an intimate person, Regina said so. Now all I want is intimacy. That's not all I need. I also want sex in my life, and I don't want the same boring sex I had with Regina." He paused for what felt like a long time.

"The whole thing is different from any other tray I have done before except the sailboat, I love the water," he added.

We both sat silently looking at the tray before the session ended.

At our next session he entered the sandplay room and said, "I don't need any mountains. I am feeling pretty good now." Then he proceeded with picking figures. He gathered the following in five miniatures: a purple non-binary couple signing a document, a miniature of Rodin's thinker, a white tiger, three non-descript figures holding hands, and a black statue of a seated cross-legged man with his head down (Figure 11.12).

"I have no idea why I picked any of these items," he said.

"I love that you just let your unconscious pick for you," I said. "That's what this is really all about."

"The black yoga figure is what I need to do to stay calm and not to get overwhelmed or stressed no matter what," he said.

He then placed his hand over the small replica of Rodin's thinker and commented, "the thinker is hoping I make good decisions." He paused.

I waited. I was curious at that moment. He talked about "the thinker" as if it was alive and held all the hope.

He continued, "the tiger is strength and confidence, the eye of the tiger." Again, I thought to myself, Billy was becoming more and more confident over the last few weeks, and I could see it in his own eyes.

He added, "the two purple figures are signing a contract. That's me meeting someone and going over the list of all the sexual things."

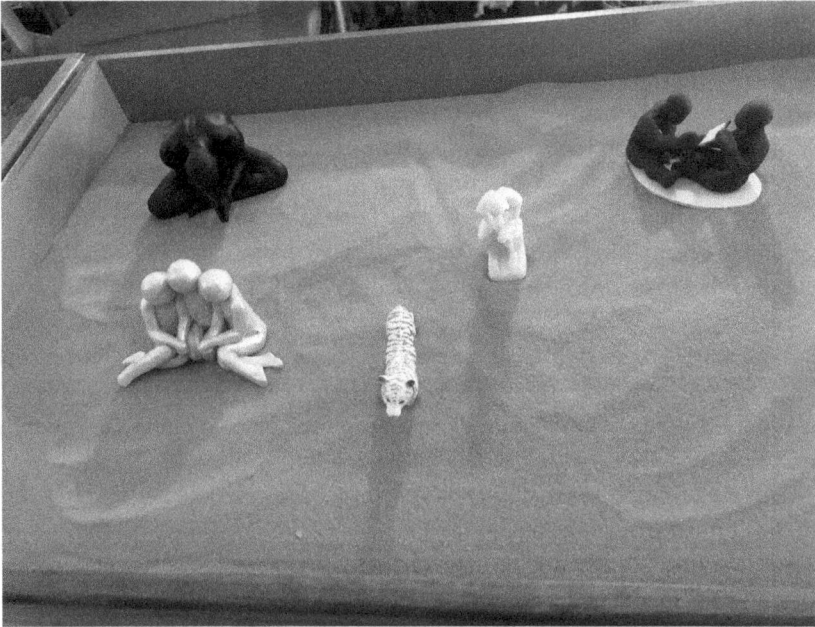

Figure 11.12 Signing a Contract

Photo by the author

I smiled at Billy, and I remembered discussing in a previous talk session how he could possibly make a bucket list of all the things he wanted in his life. This list was to include things he desired and things he found sexually pleasurable. I recalled one session when he said, "I made the list. I am now completely sure of what I want, and feel when the time is right, I will go over it with the person who can share with me their own list. It will be mutually consensual." I had been talking about the importance of consent throughout the many meetings and was happy to hear he understood the value in it.

"Whoever I am going to have a relationship with can share with me and I can learn what they want, what their limits will be, and I can freely state mine," he said while he was looking at the tray.

Billy looked into my eyes and smiled.

"Do you remember me making that list?" he asked.

"Absolutely I do," I said.

"My swinger friends..." he paused for 30 to 45 seconds. "They keep me safe."

He pointed to the three white figures on the left side of the tray.

"I had a dream about seeing my grandkids and the world was going to end" he added.

I wondered about the dream. I didn't ask him to elaborate.

"I recently saw a movie with Russell Crow where he played a gladiator. I want to be strong and have honor like him. I think of him now with integrity, and I think about that when I came clean in this therapy room with Regina. That was an honor. Our lives could have been incredible if she wanted; I was willing to do anything. I am now ready to have a partner and know I must be completely honest with them." He smiled. We ended the session.

Weeks went by and Billy did a few trays, and discussed how he was working out more to get into the best physical shape he could be in, yet he still hadn't moved any of the things his ex-wife left in her closet, and he still missed the grandchildren. At one point he said out of the blue, "Regina's last words to me were, 'If I were you, I would kill myself.'"

The next time he made a tray he came into the session and began to tell me he was thinking of dating again.

"I have to think about what type of people I want to meet. I would like to do a tray today" he said.

He selected four miniatures, three of which he had chosen before in other trays: the purple couple signing the contract, the boxer, the multi-colored couple, and a new one, a very small house (Figure 11.13).

He said, "This is me meeting someone and whipping out the list. Meeting somebody who I can discuss all sexual things with." I recognized the impact of making his sexual desires concrete and having a tool to open up about sexual play with a partner.

He continued, "the dog is companionship…being happy in my little house."

I was excited when I saw the tiny little house placed in the tray. I thought about the symbolism of houses and the possibility that this tiny house might be the beginning of Billy's finding his inner soul or Self. In addition, I felt Billy's heart was opening up to genuine and authentic intimacy. In the book, *Dictionary Dreams-Signs-Symbols: The Source Code* by Kaya, "In its global dimension, the house or apartment we live in represents our intimacy, our inner space, the place where we renew and replenish ourselves" (p. 383). Billy's house was tiny, I realized it would take time for him to fully embrace his ability to have and be an intimate person. Kalff writes, "I observed that it takes six to eight weeks until a situation made visible from the unconscious can manifest in our outer life. At the beginning it is delicate like a blade of grass just sprouted and needs careful tending" (p. 21). I was curious about how that house would transform in his sandplay series.

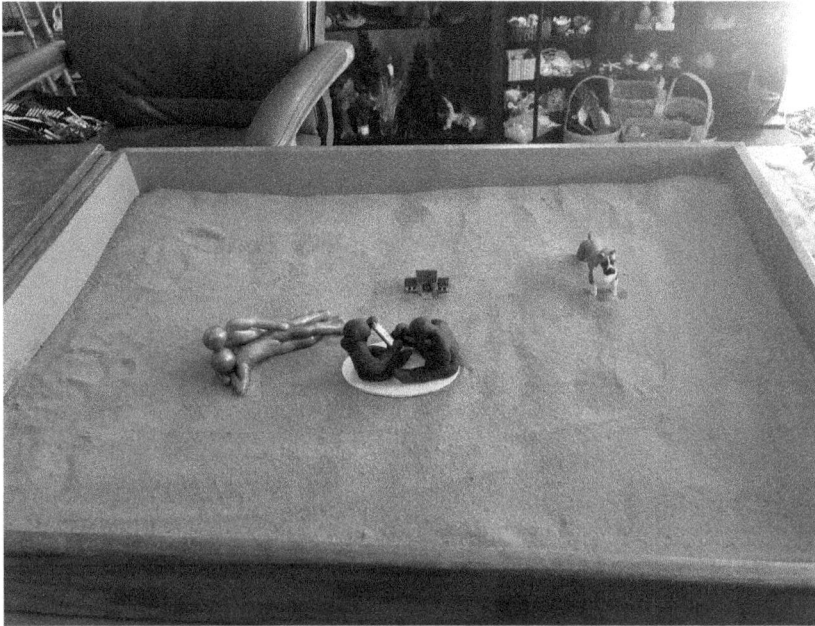

Figure 11.13 I Look at Things Differently Now
Photo by the author

In his next tray he added another symbol that suggested he was becoming stronger internally, displaying his intimacy; a bigger vessel, a large ship—to navigate the metaphorical deeper oceanic seas or emotions (Figure 11.14).

He articulated, "the white figures are me and a woman being in a relationship."

I was thrilled to see he identified himself with having intimacy for the first time he related to the couple in the tray.

Billy met a woman, Donna, a few weeks later. It was just before New Year's Eve. Approximately a week into the relationship Billy decided only to date her exclusively. When he came in for another session he said, "I haven't drunk for four weeks since I have met Donna because she is a recovering alcoholic. I am going to try to make it work with her."

Alas, three weeks later, Donna rejected him, and he reached out to a man to have sex. He said, "I drank when I met with the man, had sex, and when he left my house, I poured the rest of the Gin down the sink."

The next day Donna contacted Billy. Ironically, he made a conscious decision not to be honest with her about the sex he had with the man. They began dating again but broke up a few weeks later. He became very curious about

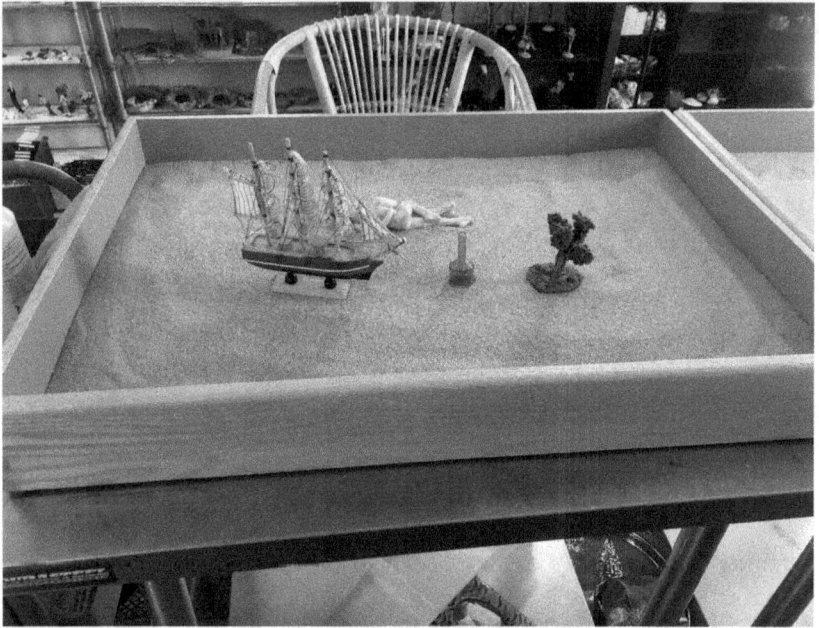

Figure 11.14 The Ship

Photo by the author

why he wasn't completely honest with Donna and wanted to understand this behavior further.

He continued with weekly appointments, shared with me how he found the therapy was working, and how he was opening up with the swingers.

"It's like the group has acted as a safe testing ground for the work we do at your office," he said. "Now it's moving into my private dating life."

Billy met another woman, Phyllis, whom he dated for about three and a half weeks before they ended the relationship. It was approximately one month later when he came into a session excited. I wondered what was happening in his life. He told me he met a woman named Halley through a blind date set up by a friend.

"I was introduced to her, and we had talked on the phone for three hours and twenty minutes last Friday. She came to my house on Sunday. This was the first time I met her in person. She came up the stairs onto my porch and we just looked at each other. Within five minutes we were passionately kissing each other."

He told me he didn't understand exactly how the kiss happened. They went for a hike, came back to his house, talked for hours, and things got pretty hot. He said he didn't want to have sex with Halley without telling her everything he has been doing and wanted her to know all of it. He said he told her everything about his sexual desires, having sex with men, and what happened between Regina and himself. He told Halley how much he still missed Regina's daughter Janet and her children whom he considered his grandchildren. He also said Halley was very sheltered when it came to sex, and they talked for a long time about the subject.

"I feel incredible and will not be devastated if it doesn't work out. I had no expectations, never expected for all of that to happen so fast and I was completely open with her." Before I could say a word, he added, "So I think I am getting better. I will know by Thursday for sure."

I smiled at his vivacity and exuberance. "Holy cow Billy, that's a lot of information. It sounds like you were upfront and feel good about that."

"I do Peg, I feel like she will be okay with anything I tell her, and I feel we have chemistry like no one I have ever been with before. Not even Regina. Peg, I have to tell you now, I stopped feeling shame about anal sex. You helped me explore my subconscious and past to discover why I liked anal sex. This led to me discovering the events in my life that made me feel shame. I could not figure out why I liked anal sex and was not attracted to men just the sex. Although, I had sex with men to fill my cravings, mainly because men were easily available and most of them were married like me at the time, and wanted the same thing."

He added, "You helped me understand the events in my life that were difficult for me, these events included my dad not liking gay people, how I had anal sex and blowjobs with other boys from the age of six to twelve while I was growing up, being exposed to large amounts of sex magazines, and sex storybooks at the age of ten."

"While working with you Peg, I started to believe that there was nothing wrong with what I liked. If I was honest with myself and others, consensual, I should pursue what I liked. The shame has gone away. Somewhere along the line, I stopped worrying about others finding out about my liking anal sex. I have come to realize that for me to have a great relationship with someone they must be willing to please me in that way or it just won't work out for the long run. I also think the art project we did about my problems, successes, and failures has contributed to the end of my shame."

The session came to an end, and I was exhilarated. Billy had changed. I couldn't wait to see him again. I knew he would only require a few more sessions with me. He came in a few weeks later and did a sandplay tray.

When asked about his sandplay world he stated, "just me finding love, hanging out with Halley, just enjoying each other's company. We were recently watching a hallmark movie and she said, 'That kind of love isn't real.'

"I used to say that, and now I know it is real" I said to her.

"You know I feel honest, open with Halley, and it just feels right. She is totally opposite of the type of woman I would go with before, she's a little overweight, and she has such a mellow personality. This is what this tray is about."

Billy shared his feelings about his tray. I recognized how different this was from the first tray he had competed about 12 months ago, the one earlier with the mountains. I noticed the house was in the same hues, the white and gray, and black mountains, and it wasn't small like the last house he put in his tray. I thought this looked like a home more than just a four-walled structure. Also, the woman in the tray was entirely different from any other feminine figure he had put in the sand. She was not thin-waisted with big breasts like the yoga figure, and she was much more rounded. She appeared comfortable with her body wearing a two-piece swimsuit and a brimmed hat. I was also delighted to see the tree return. Billy seemed to be accessing more of his own Self-energy. The sailboat was still the vehicle of choice in navigating his emotional ocean. I loved seeing the little steps visually connecting the woman with the home. It seemed the unconscious was saying, "take baby steps" (Figure 11.15).

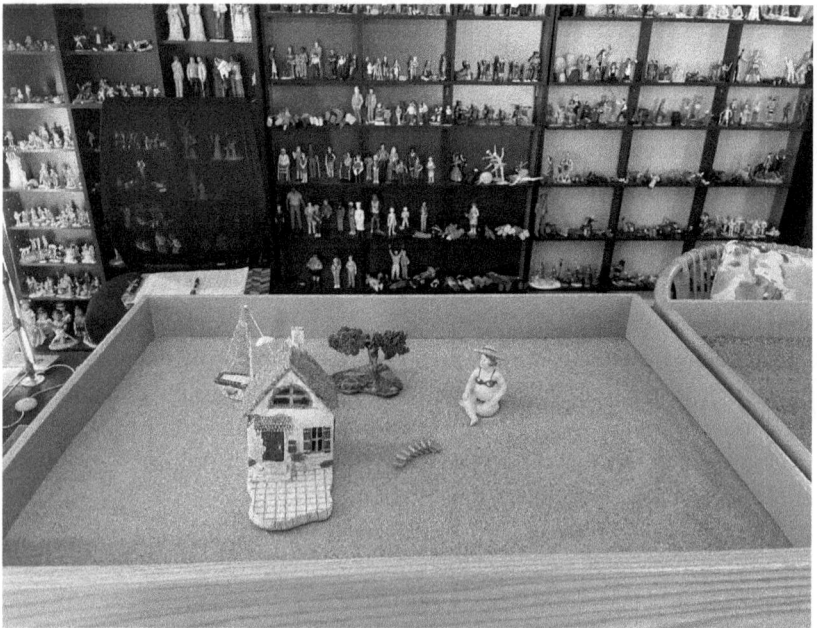

Figure 11.15 Smalls Steps

Photo by the author

He shared, "I am ashamed of what I did to my ex-wife, we could have had the hallmark thing, and with Halley I haven't wanted anal sex. This time is different. We're not so concerned about the sex stuff, and we get along so well. We'll see what happens."

"Is there more you would like to share?" I asked.

He immediately sat back in his chair, smiled like the Cheshire Cat in *Alice in Wonderland*, and his eyes were beaming. "I thought you would never ask! I am so very happy to have met Halley. I think she is my girlfriend now. I get so turned on by her even though she is heavier than I am used to. We had anal sex and she loved it. She was also very curious about my anal toys and even wanted to use them on me. Over the weekend we went to dinner with one of the swinger couples, and she thought they were so nice. Halley and I are having sex a few times a night, and I think it's great. We are even going to buy a strap-on for her to play with me."

I was overjoyed to hear how his life was changing and said, "This is so great to hear how happy you are." Then I asked, "Is there more you'd like to say?"

"Hell yeah!" he replied. "I know the swinger group is my safety net and I don't want to leave them yet—or maybe at all. And another thing: I realized I wasn't honest with my ex-wife and now I am completely straight-forward with Halley. She knows everything, I didn't hold back one little secret, I even told her about the fisting I did with the gay guy, and she even knows I see you!"

Billy, this is amazing. It seems like you're a completely different man." I replied.

"I know, I have never been this happy, things are going great, I haven't told Halley I love her, and I know she's in love with me. We went to a concert, she had a fantastic time, and she just about said it. I know she's waiting for me to say it first. I just want to be sure; I need to meet her kids."

A couple of weeks passed before Billy came in for his next sandplay session. He walked into the room, appearing content and at ease. We chatted for a few moments, and he told me he wasn't suffering from loneliness any longer. He still felt emotionally vulnerable and admitted to watching *Gladiator* again: he even cried when Russell Crow's character died. I appreciated Billy at that moment. He was showing a quality of compassion for others.

When he entered the sandplay room he walked around for approximately 20 minutes. He moved from shelf to shelf, wall by wall, and couldn't seem to find any miniatures. He looked over to me at least four times. I made eye contact and smiled back at him. He continued searching the shelves, stopped at the tree section, and picked up a red-leaf tree. He turned and looked at

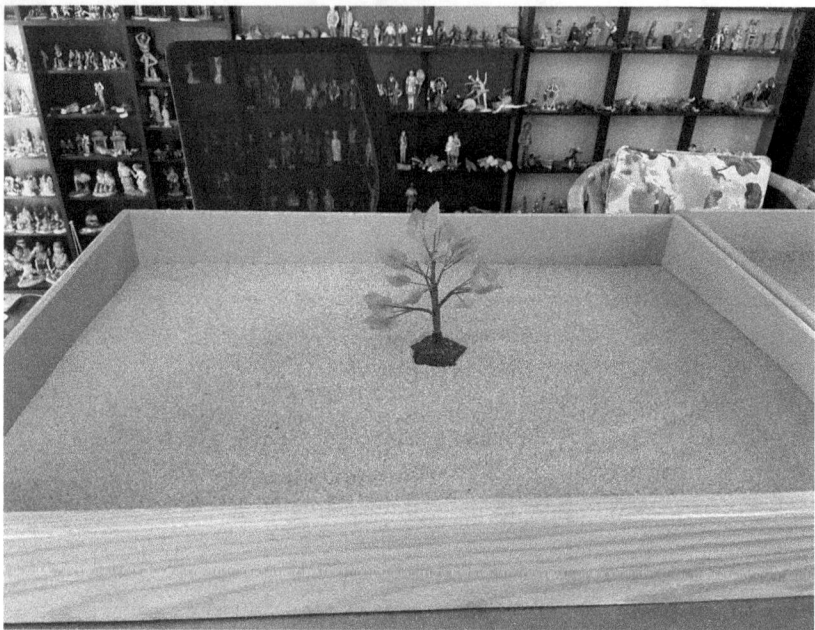

Figure 11.16 Red Tree

Photo by the author

me, I nodded my head, and he stood before the dry sand tray. He placed the brightly colored tree in the center of the tray (Figure 11.16).

"It feels like a new start," he said, stepping back to look at the tray. "I don't feel any baggage or anything like I did when I first started therapy with you. I don't have any secrets, I guess it has to do with Halley, I am living authentically and with directness."

I waited a few moments and he spoke again.

"I have to tell you the first thing Halley and I might do at the next swinger's party is have sex with another man. She has been watching sexual imagery with two men and told me she is ready to explore this." He laughed out loud and added, "she was so vanilla prior to meeting me."

I laughed too and added, "Billy it's funny how now you use the word, 'vanilla.' When you came in for your initial session, you never would have said anything like that. It's exciting to see how much you have learned, including acceptance of yourself. I am so pleased to have been on this journey with you."

I looked at the single red tree and realized this was a transformative tray for Billy. He now had a sense of himself, and the tray felt special to me. This was typical of a tree located in New England in the fall, when the colors are magnificent, and the sun brightly shines down to warm the earth when the temperatures grow cooler. Billy's true distinctive personality, with all its unique qualities, was in the center of that tray. It was a profound tray; it was truly enlightening.

Two weeks later Billy did his last tray with me, although neither Billy nor I knew this at the time he walked into the sandplay room.

"I have to tell you something and this time you really are going to be surprised," he said. His face radiated dynamism.

"Okay, I am ready for it," I said enthusiastically.

"I told Halley I loved her!"

"You're kidding. I love that!"

"No, I am not kidding," he said. "I just couldn't wait another minute and had to tell her." "What happened that you couldn't wait?" I asked.

"Remember I met her little grandchild on her boat a while back?" he asked. "Well, it was his second birthday and Halley invited me over to celebrate. I had so much fun with Halley. Her daughter hugged me and said, 'It's so nice to see you again.' I have something else to tell you. Halley is going to take off her acrylic nails that she has had for years. I never expected that."

I wasn't sure what the significance of the nails was, exactly and why it was bringing him joy. I was going to ask him when he interrupted. "Okay, now I can do a tray." He walked towards the shelf, and, like the last time, he seemed perplexed. He turned to me and said, "I have no idea what I am going to pick today."

"Just see what comes to you," I said.

A few minutes later he quickly picked a tree, walked directly to where the bridges are stored, and swiftly crossed the room to where a family statue was located. He grabbed it and began placing the miniatures in the tray.

When all three symbols were positioned, I asked him if it was complete, and he confirmed it was. I immediately looked at the upside-down bridge and felt my heart drop. I couldn't understand. Bridges are significant for connection. It appeared he deliberately placed it the wrong way. I was confused and saddened (Figure 11.17).

"Does the tray feel complete?" I asked.

"Yes," Billy said.

He began telling me about his tray with tears streaming down his face. "I guess the tree is happiness. The bridge is upside-down because it's gone."

I was now feeling my own stomach turn inside out.

"I've crossed that bridge. I'm done. It had to be upside down. I don't understand why I picked the family. Maybe it's the old family, or maybe it's a new one coming. I just don't know what the angel is or what that one means."

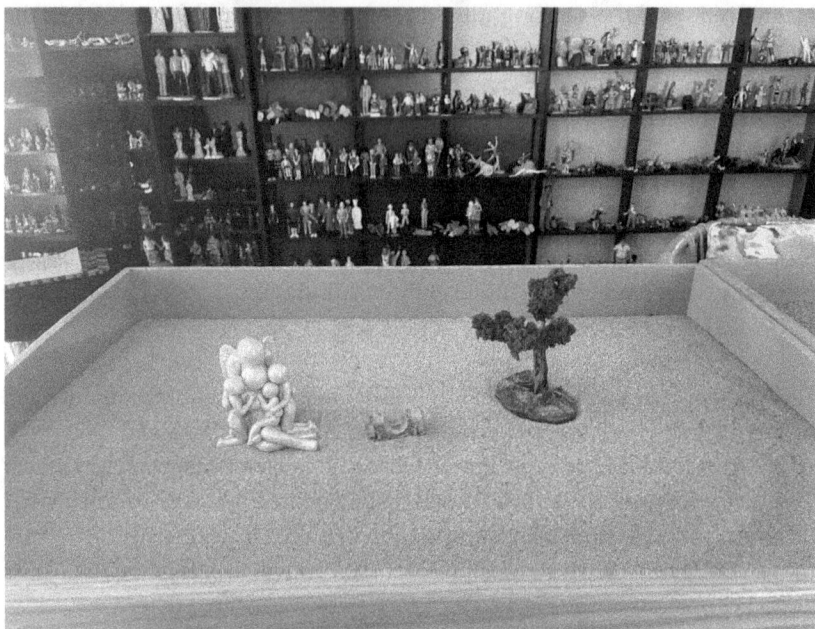

Figure 11.17 The Upside-Down Bridge

Photo by the author

I remained quiet, and he continued.

"I thought about that bridge being upside-down and I knew it needed to be flipped. I don't need a bridge anymore. I have made it to the point where I am now connected to Halley and myself."

I began to tear up because I had never seen anyone ever put a bridge upside-down before, and I assumed it was bad. To Billy, the bridge was no longer needed. It was GREAT! Billy had made the transition to a place of internal peace. This is what he and most people truly desired. I looked at him and shook my head back and forth, grabbing a tissue. We both smiled at each other, and I think we both knew he had completed his sandplay process.

Two weeks later we met for our final session. I loved his departing words.

"Oh, I forgot to mention. Halley fisted me on Sunday. There wasn't any drinking, drugs, poppers, or anything. Her fist went in easier than ever. When her hand went in, she got so emotional and almost cried because she knew how important a moment it was for me. She also told me she liked doing it. We both couldn't believe it."

This made me smile because I finally understood the significance of Halley removing her acrylic nails. She, too, was letting go of something so she could help Billy experiment with his sexual desires without adding the risk of injury. Something that had previously brought him shame was now out in the open, and both partners could share in the experience without fear of judgment and condemnation.

After we finished up the sessions and said our goodbyes, he paused at the door and smiled at me. A year later I called Billy to see how he was doing. He and Halley were still together. She had met and enjoyed being with all his swinger friends, and I loved the metaphor he said to me to describe how I helped him.

He said, "Peg, thank you for all your help. When we ended our sessions I had training wheels, now I am riding the bicycle without them, and now that I don't have to live with all the shame, I have been experiencing healthy relationships with people. I notice I am going through life with calmness, clarity, and I am connecting with others. Thank you."

Resources

Bradway, K., "Transference and countertransference in sandplay therapy," *Journal of Sandplay Therapy*, 1(1), 1991, p. 29.

Cozolino, L., *The neuroscience of human relationships: Attachment and the developing social brain*. W. W. Norton & Company, New York, NY, 2014 (pp. 249–250).

Dana, D., *The polyvagal theory in therapy: Engaging the rhythm of regulation*. W. W. Norton & Company, New York, NY, 2018 (p. 44).

Freedle, L., "Healing trauma through sandplay: A neuropsychological perspective," *The Routledge international handbook of sandplay therapy*. Routledge, New York, NY, 2017 (pp. 190–205).

Jung, C. G., *The practice of psychotherapy, the psychology of the transference*, CW16 p. 249. Bollingen Foundation Published by Princeton University Press, Princeton, NJ, 1985 (Original Copyright 1954).

Kalff, D. M., *Sandplay: A psychotherapeutic approach to the psyche* (B. L. Matthews, Trans.). Analytical Psychology Press, Oberlin, OH, Sandplay Edition: 3rd ed., 2020 (Original work published 1966) (pp. 5, 21, 103).

Kalsched, D., *Trauma and the soul: A psycho-spiritual approach to human development and its interruption*. Routledge, New York, NY, 2013 (p. 20).

Kaya, *Dictionary. Dreams-signs-symbols: The source code*. Universe/City Mikael, Non-profit organization. Publishing House, Canada, 2013 (p. 383).

Porges, S., Polyvagal theory: A biobehavioral journey to sociality. *Comprehensive Psychoneuroendocrinology*, 7, 2021, p. 100069. https://doi.org/10.1016/j.cpnec.2021.100069.

Rediger, J., *Cured: The life-changing science of spontaneous healing*. Flatiron Books, New York, NY, 2020 (p. 193).

Jane

12

Letting Go of Painful Sex Through IFSsandtray

Jane, a client who emailed me hoping to find another way to heal from vaginismus, wrote,

> I have been looking into working with a sex therapist and was impressed with your website and experience. I am a 56-year-old woman, and my goal is to have a healthy sex life though middle age and beyond. I struggle with PTSD, vaginismus, confusion and shame over sexual identity, depression, and anxiety. I have done EMDR in the past and now I am motivated and hopeful that working with you will improve my quality of life!

When I read Jane's email, I thought there was a high probability, like many of my clients, that she never had the opportunity to experience a form of therapy that taps into the power of the unconscious mind. I found myself drawn to Jane's willingness and enthusiasm which have always been good indications of someone prepared to try uniquely different therapeutic techniques which I was offering.

Some of my colleagues who studied with me in advanced training have told their clients, "I have been in a new training and learned something completely unlike anything we have been doing, would you be willing to try it?" Most have said their clients respond in the affirmative. This is often what I have done in my therapeutic practice.

When I met Jane for the first time I was immediately impressed with her sense of style, the way she moved so confidently across the room, and how

DOI: 10.4324/9781003388302-14

powerful and strong she appeared in her relatively small-framed, slim body. I could tell she was a person who had some sense of positive self-esteem by how she carried herself. She was impeccably dressed in designer shoes, carried a high-end handbag, and had a very stylish haircut.

Once Jane was seated, I asked her to just take a moment to settle into the space. I informed her that I did this with every client because it's important for the autonomic nervous system. When she looked at me quizzically, I said, "I will explain more about that in a few minutes." I watched as she took a deep breath, slowly gazed around the room, looked at the various books on the bookshelf, looked me in the eye, and began to talk.

"I decided to see you for therapy because I know that I will not be able to have the type of relationship I want with myself and a significant other if I don't address my sexual issues. I had been to sex therapy in the past with partners, first with my husband, then with my girlfriend who became my significant other. In those sessions, I hated being the person who was 'broken and needed to be fixed.' This time I want it to be different—to do it for myself only. I want to reclaim my sexuality."

"Jane I am so glad you are here and shared that with me. Is there more?"

Asking an open-ended question like "Is there more?" Often eases any residual tension and allows the client to go a little deeper. At this point, I am certain to listen carefully, and watch for signs of what the body may be experiencing such as any forms of tension or relaxation, and I become curious.

"I had pain during sex with my ex-husband, and during gynecological exams," she said. "That may have been a reason why I pursued a relationship with a woman after my marriage dissolved. After the relationship with the woman ended, my doctor and I talked about whether I could ever have sex with a man—that I was too small and had atrophy. I was diagnosed with vaginismus."

She then added, "I studied psychology in college. I am a little skeptical and wondered if any therapist is ever going to be able to help me. I don't want to be in therapy forever. I am only committing to five sessions unless I see your nontraditional treatment methods are different from all of the previous therapists who just talk to me."

"I completely get why you are skeptical given your history with therapists," I said. "I do work differently. I am going to explain some of that to you now and after that, I am going to ask you if you would like to try an experiment. Let's first start with clarifying what I said a little earlier about why I had you just sit for a few moments in order to have your autonomic nervous system adjust to this office."

Jane and I took a few minutes chatting about the body and mind, the basics of the Polyvagal Theory (PVT), and concepts found in the Internal Family Systems (IFS) model, how everyone has Parts, and the various ways I work with sand. To simplify this complex concept, I discussed how the body and mind work together and cannot be separated. In therapy, both have to be considered in the treatment. I then asked if she was ready to try the experiment. She enthusiastically agreed and said, "I know you work differently, and I am willing to try anything."

I reached over to one of the two sets of 3-by-5-inch laminated Pro-Symptom Belief Cards (see chapter eight," How Beliefs Influence Therapy: Introduction to The Pro-Symptom Belief Cards) that I keep on the end table to my left.

I asked Jane to choose the cards she felt were true about herself whenever she thought about having sex. She selected about ten. I then asked her to find the one card that felt the truest to her out of these, and she selected, "it's not okay to show or feel my emotions."

In his book, *"Cured: The Life-Changing Science of Spontaneous Healing,"* Dr. Jeffrey Rediger explains how negative viewpoints are held in the brain and are called "default mode networks." He writes, "And the great thing about the term *default mode network* [DMN] is that it accurately captures the way that identity is a function of neural synapses and pathways that can be edited or redrawn, the way a map can be edited or redrawn as a landscape changes over time" (p. 276). He further writes, "When you get out of the DMN, you have the chance to create and reinforce new neural pathways that can override existing ones" (p. 276). When I first read this, I was excited because now it all made sense to me. The healing I witness while using sand with my clients has changed the old neural pathway to a new one.

The cards were designed specifically to represent Protectors, both Managers and Firefighters in the modality Internal Family Systems (IFS). For more clarity about Parts in therapy (see Chapter 5, "Multiplicity: Introduction to Parts in Therapy) gain a better comprehension of how all Parts, including Protectors, relate to the autonomic nervous system.

I asked Jane if she wanted to go further in possibly finding out where this belief stemmed from. "Absolutely," she replied. I asked her if she felt safe to close her eyes, explaining how we were going to focus on her body. If she didn't feel safe, she didn't have to close them and could do the experiment with her eyes open. In addition, I explained that what we were about to do would address feelings and beliefs held in her body. All the visual stimulation of being in a new space might make it more difficult to focus internally because of the unfamiliarity.

She closed her eyes. I asked her to focus on where she felt it wasn't okay to show or feel her emotions in her body. The combination of techniques—Sensorimotor Psychotherapy, which focuses on the body, and IFS, focusing on the Parts of Jane's system, and the belief—enabled her to recall a few upsetting memories. These beliefs usually are held by Parts that are younger than five.

One of the earliest memories Jane shared occurred when she was very young. She saw a scene in her mind's eye of a time when she was playing with her father. They were having fun together, and out of nowhere, he began yelling at her. She recalled feeling extremely scared and felt sick to her stomach. I asked Jane how she was doing, and she said she was okay, and I asked her to follow that memory back further by focusing on the Part's body. She couldn't go back any younger. I then asked her to open her eyes, and she said to me, "That was powerful. I had forgotten all about that. I now remember it—when it happened. I think I was around four." We had a few more minutes left in the session, and we processed what had just happened. When the session ended Jane was inspired and left feeling a sense of hope. We scheduled the next session for two weeks later.

During the next session, Jane informed me she was spiritual but not religious, single, and in a relationship with a man she loved and respected. She described him as loyal, easy-going, calm, and a "super nice guy." She also said he was patient and knew about her vaginismus and was attuned to her needs. She said she questioned her sexual orientation all her life, had a history of PTSD, and tried medication a few times in the past but wasn't currently on anything now. She also told me she suffered from ongoing back problems.

When I asked her to share about upsetting events in her life, she told me she had been sexually and emotionally abused by her father when she was young. Her father's brother groped her when she was a little girl, and there was a lot of sexual inappropriateness throughout her childhood. She informed me when she was very young, her mother would hurt her whenever she washed Jane's genitals.

She discussed her college years. She had an experience with a man that was non-consensual, and she said, "I can't call it rape because he came on my stomach." Jane spoke about having difficulty with fertility when she and her husband were trying to conceive. They adopted two children; she divorced him many years ago when the kids were younger. She then had a relationship with a woman for four years and now she was in a loving relationship with her significant other, David. She said, "When I started a relationship with David, we had a long discussion about my concern that we may never be able to have intercourse. This did not matter to him, which took some of the pressure off me."

Now that I had a better understanding of Jane's needs, I told her we would be working with the sand and miniatures in our next session.

When Jane arrived for her third visit and we settled in the meeting space for a few minutes. I checked in with her to see how she was feeling and if she had anything on her agenda that she wanted to address. She said, "No, I am looking forward to working with the sand."

We entered the sandplay room and Jane appeared excited and ready to engage. I recalled our first meeting when she said she was skeptical, so I kept that in mind. This was going to be a very different type of therapy for her, and I wondered if her skeptical Part was going to show up in today's session. If it did, I knew how to handle it. I have experienced skeptical, suspicious, and questioning Parts before. All Parts have a positive intention for the client; they are there to make sure the client isn't deceived. Their job is to protect the individual and often just want to understand what is happening. Jane sat before the tray with dry sand, didn't touch the sand, and looked at me with a quizzical face. Her face softened as I explained what to expect.

"Jane, what we are going to do today is work with the miniatures in the sand. This is strongly based in the modality of Internal Family Systems. I call this IFSsandtray. There are basically two ways I work with the sand. One is what we are going to do today where I will ask you to find a figure on the shelves to represent the Part of you that is most likely protecting you from having sex with your partner. The other way I work with sand is called sandplay. When we do a sandplay session, that will be 180 degrees unlike what we do today. Sandplay is nondirective, whereas IFSsandtray is very directive. I think you will end up doing both, each one works equally well. Does that make sense so far?"

"I think so," she said. "If I have any questions, is it okay if I ask you?"

"That's an unequivocal yes," I said. "Just ask away. I am only going to work at the pace that works best for you."

She took a deep breath.

"Are you ready to begin?" I asked.

"Yes."

"Fabulous. The first thing I want you to do is find a miniature from anywhere on the shelves to represent the Part of you that is giving you pain with sex."

She got up from her chair and began looking at the shelves behind her—an entire wall of human figures. She looked at them carefully, touched and picked up two, put them back on the shelf, and then found a 5-inch-tall figurine of a woman dressed in a black leather studded bra and panties, white fringed black leather boots with matching leather elbow-length fingerless gloves or cuffs, black chaps, and she held a gun in her right hand. It appeared the figure had its finger on the trigger. Jane came back to her seat, placed the miniature into the tray facing herself, and then looked up at me (Figure 12.1).

I looked at the figure, immediately recognizing how much it reminded me of Jane. It had presence, its own style, and meant business. I was curious

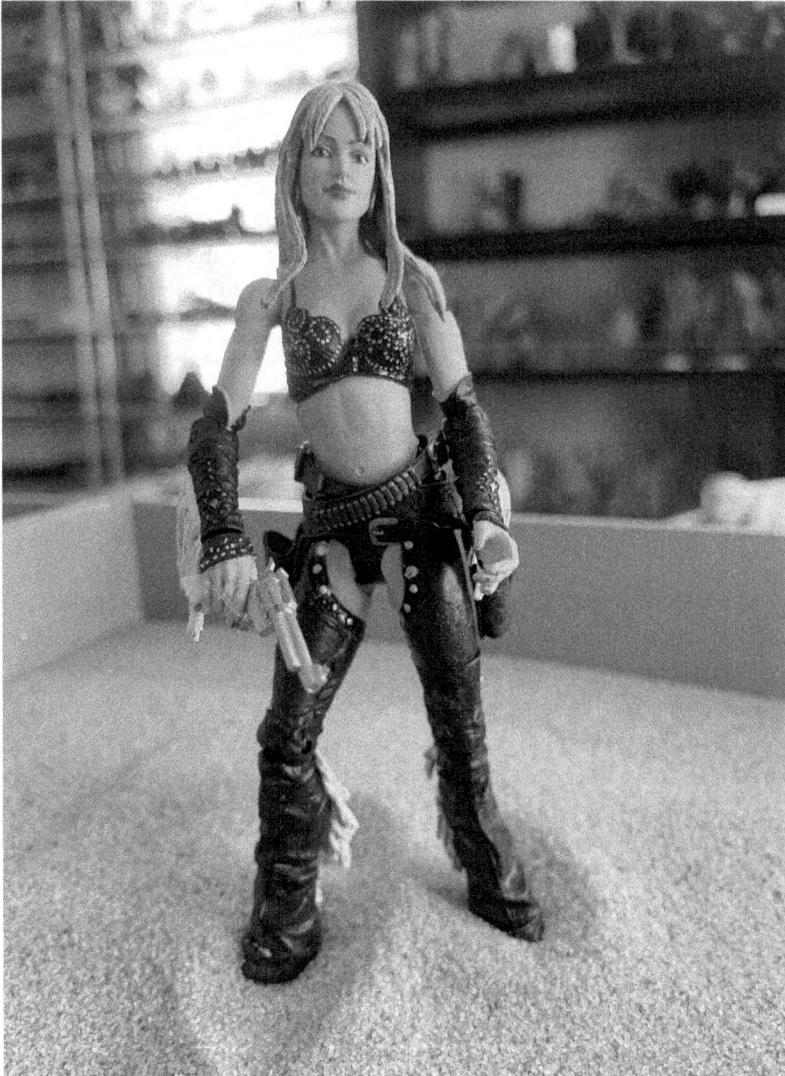

Figure 12.1 Miniature Dressed in Black Leather

Photo by the author

about what was going to happen in the next 30 minutes, recalling how Jane wanted results in five sessions.

"Jane, thanks for finding her," I said. "She stands in the tray before you, I wonder how you feel towards her?"

"I hate her," she replied.

I thought she was going to say that. Many people, like Jane, hate their Parts because they don't know they are trying to protect them. In this case I was certain the figure in the tray was a Firefighter in the IFS model. The Firefighter is a protector that always tries to avoid the feelings of emotional pain held by the Exile. In the person's mind, the Exile is the Part that carries the original wound. In Jane's case this may have been the Part reacting to the unwanted touching from her uncle and the sexual abuse by her father. Other Exiles in a person's system can stem from early childhood neglect, mis-attunement from the caregivers, and any form of physical or emotional abuse. The Firefighter Part will compel the individual to do anything to avoid feeling the emotional pain from that original wound.

At that moment I had to decide how I wanted Jane to meet the very Part of her that helped her survive her early childhood sexual abuse from her father. It most likely developed at the time of the abuse. There are various ways I might convey this idea in IFSsandtray. This time I choose to use a technique I learned in my IFS training. I was going to talk directly to the miniature, which represented the Protector Part of Jane that now was externalized in front of us.

"Jane, what I am about to do isn't going to make any logical sense to you. I think it's going to be profound. Are you interested in learning more about this Part of you that we see before us now?"

"Sure," she said. "I know you work in a different way, and I am ready."

"Okay, what I am about to do is talk directly to this Part of you and I am going to ask it questions. What I want you to do is say the first thing that you think—and don't edit. Some of these thoughts may not make any sense to you. I want you to just say them out loud. They will make sense to me. Any questions?"

"You want me to just say the first thing that comes to my mind, right? I certainly can do that."

"Okay, I am now going to talk directly to the figure." I paused, bent over so I was at eye level with the miniature, and began.

"Hi woman in the tray. I see you, and I love how you are dressed all in leather. I don't have any leather on today, but I too love leather, and wear it in the winter. I would love to get to know you a little bit if that would be okay with you. My name is Peg." As I talked, I tilted my head to the right purposely to show her I was curious and interested in her, a separate entity from Jane. I knew she was looking at everything I was doing through Jane's eyes and hearing every word I was saying through Jane's ears. It was imperative for me to let her know I saw her individually as a Part of Jane and not Jane who was sitting in front of me. In addressing the figure directly, it allows the Part of Jane that is externalized in the sand to know it is separate from Jane. It has now taken on a physical form as the figurine and has its own identity.

When I work with any clients with skeptical Parts which are protective Parts, they might say things like this is silly or embarrassing. When that happens, I will often check in with the client, ask for permission to look into their eyes, and address the concerns of the Part. This is always done from a place within me that is truly curious. The curious aspect of myself is called Self in Internal Family Systems. This technique is known as direct access.

In his book, *No Bad Parts* written in 2021, Dr. Richard Schwartz wrote, "… there was a point where I talked directly to the protector, a practice we call *direct access*" (p. 46). This method of communication allows the clinician to have a dialog with the Part. This is exactly what Dr. Schwartz addressed in many of the books he has written.

I continued, "I know Jane just said she doesn't like you. I know she just doesn't understand you yet. I think by the end of this meeting she will. I wonder if it would be okay if I ask you a few questions? I am going to look at Jane for a quick second and let her know you are going to speak through her mouth if you choose." At that moment I moved my body upward, looked Jane in the eyes, and asked, "Would you mind if she uses your mouth to speak to me?"

Jane looked at me for a moment, paused, and then said, "Yes. Of course."

"Thanks Jane, now I want you to just say the first thing that comes to your mind and remember don't edit anything even if it doesn't make sense to you. Okay?"

"Okay" she replied.

I bent back over to be eye level with the miniature, tilted my head in curiosity again, looked directly at the figure and began. "Thanks for letting me talk to Jane. She just agreed you can speak through her mouth. I look forward to hearing what you have to say. Can I ask you a few questions now?"

"Yes," I heard in Jane's voice.

"Thanks, first I am wondering if you have a name or how should I address you?"

"BITCH" I heard Jane say out loud in an angry voice.

I knew immediately I had connected to the Part inside of Jane that was trying to help her in some way. She wanted to be called Bitch. I also knew

I had to match Bitch's emotional intensity for it to recognize I was taking her seriously, so I raised my voice, changed my tone to reflect that I could meet her on her level, and I could work on her trusting me to handle everything she was about to tell me.

"So, your name is BITCH, do I have that right?"

"Yeah, you got that right," Bitch said.

I quickly looked up at Jane, saw she had her eyes wide open as if she couldn't believe what just happened. I made eye contact with her, nodded my head, and continued with my conversation with Bitch.

"Bitch, I wonder what's your job in Jane's system?"

"I fucking protect that piece of shit," Bitch said.

I immediately knew I was talking to Jane's Firefighter. I liked and respected Bitch very much. I understood she probably called Jane a piece of shit because she knew Jane had another Part that hated her.

I asked Jane in the beginning of the session how she felt toward the Part and she said she hated it. In knew in this moment this wasn't Jane in Self talking but rather another Part talking. I knew this and wasn't worried, so I continued.

"Bitch how long have you had your job?"

"Forever." Bitch replied.

"I wonder, how old was Jane when you took on your job?"

"She was about three," Bitch replied.

"How old are you?"

"Seven," she said.

"Bitch, how do you protect Jane?"

"I shut her down. I shut her down sexually, mentally, and physically. I am very angry!" Bitch said.

"What are you so angry about?"

"I am angry because Jane betrayed me," Bitch said.

"How did she betray you?"

"She doesn't listen to me. After all I have done for her. She ignores me. I NEVER GET HEARD!" Bitch replied in an angry tone. It seemed she was filled with rage.

"Hmmm, that's got to be very difficult for you when Jane doesn't listen to you, do I have that right?" I asked.

"Yes, you got it," Bitch said in a less angry voice. I felt compassion for her. She added, "Jane tries to bargain with me, and I hate that. I just want to shoot genitalia—penises specifically. Jane is stupid and NOT heeding my warnings. No one can be trusted. Men suck. I am not going to let Jane be a vulnerable idiot. I need to be heard, respected, and appreciated."

"Yeah, Bitch I totally get what you are saying. Makes perfect sense to me. Would you mind if I talk to Jane now, just for a minute or so to see if she understood what you are saying. Would that be all right?"

"Sure. Go right ahead," Bitch said in a calm voice.

I straightened my back, looked up at Jane who was still staring at the miniature. I waited for a few seconds before I spoke again. Jane looked me in the eyes, and I looked back directly into hers, knowing Bitch was watching me.

"Jane, did you just hear Bitch tell me how she has been protecting you?"

She took a deep breath and said, "Yes, I heard every word. I get it now. I didn't realize she was protecting me. I wonder how I can let her know I do appreciate her."

"Jane, you can send her that message now, just look at her, and tell her."

"Bitch, I am so sorry I have neglected to hear you," Jane said, addressing the figure directly. "I am so sorry. I will try to do better."

"I promised Bitch I would only check in with you for a minute. Would you mind if I check back in with her and see if she heard you?" I asked. Jane nodded her head yes. "Bitch did you hear Jane?" I asked.

"Yes, I did," Bitch said.

"I am going to ask Jane to check in with you for the next couple of days. Would that be okay with you?"

"Yes," she replied.

"Jane, I think it's important that you start to have dialogues with Bitch. Does that make sense to you?

"Absolutely," Jane said. "I am going to talk with her from now on."

After that session Jane said, "This sand therapy is really weird, but it seems to work. Can I schedule weekly appointments?"

As a result of that session with Bitch, Jane learned to send appreciation to, listen to, and talk to Bitch whenever she and David were going to become sexually intimate. I expressed to Jane that she may want to have an internal dialogue or conversation with Bitch the next time she wanted to have sex with David.

Despite Jane's initial caveat that she would only attend five sessions to see if she trusted the process, she continued seeing me well beyond that. At our 11th session, Jane reported, "Since that session when you talked to Bitch, I now have learned to respect her, I talk to her every time David and I want to make love. I had sex five times in the last two weeks since, and it was fabulous. Unfortunately, when I got drunk one of the times, I didn't talk to her, and David wasn't able to penetrate me."

I've come to understand how externalizing Parts in the sand often makes it easier for clients to see their Parts. These Parts have been working diligently behind the scenes for years and years. They always have positive intentions. Once they feel heard and gain a sense of connection with the individual, they can and will heal. I have been using this technique several times a week over the years and still can't believe how effective it is. By addressing the Protector's concerns, giving them a voice, and listening to what they say, they will give access to the wounded exile and the client will heal.

Jane　　　　　　　　　　　　　　13

Polarization of Shame and Being Sexually Free

In Chapter 12 you met Jane for the first time. This chapter expands on Jane's treatment of being a sexual being, struggling with deeply rooted shame, and how two opposite emotions, known as Parts in the Internal Family Systems (IFS) model work to protect her. Each of these Parts is known as Protectors in IFS, each having positive intentions to help Jane but reacting in entirely different ways. This is known as polarization.

It was a Tuesday morning and I looked at my schedule happy to see who I was going to see that day. At 10 am, I opened the door to the waiting room and greeted Jane. I invited her into the inner office, and she sat down and began her weekly check-in. Jane informed me that she noticed she was having an emotional reaction to something that happened three days prior. She and her partner David were at her home in her bedroom making love, late Sunday afternoon. She unexpectedly heard the back door to the mudroom open and close and knew it was her 18-year-old son coming home earlier than he usually does on a Sunday. Moments later she became distraught and shut down. She was upset and felt shameful because her son may have heard them.

"I don't know why I have been unable to process this or feel a sense of shame, it's been three days," she said. "I know my son couldn't hear anything; we were upstairs, and he was downstairs near the kitchen when he came in. There's no way he could have heard anything. This is completely illogical."

"Jane, emotional responses are Parts, and they don't know or understand logic," I reminded her. "This is your autonomic nervous system sensing something was dangerous. The shame you have is linked with other events

DOI: 10.4324/9781003388302-15

in your life that made you feel shame. Shame is not something we are born with, it's something we feel due to what happens to us, from others who judge or make us feel terrible about what we have done. It's not about what happened on Sunday when your son walked into the house, and I know it feels like it is. Would you like to work on that today or do you have anything else that you might like to focus on?"

"No, I really want to work on this today because in my mind I didn't do anything wrong and don't understand why I am feeling shameful," she said.

"Okay, what I think is happening is you have two Parts that are polarized. One that feels shameful and the other that feels you didn't do anything wrong. Do I have that right?"

"Yes, that's it exactly," she said.

"Jane, I know you have done EMDR (Eye Movement Desensitization Reprocessing) before. Today I'd like to process both Parts using IFSsandtray combining EMDR. Will that be okay with you?"

"Yes," she said. "I trust you. Let's do that."

"Another reason why EMDR will work is the boundaries created by the size of the tray. The tray has been designed so you can view the whole of what you placed inside without moving your head. I am an EMDR therapist. I have found this helpful to externalize the Parts in the sand, place them on opposite sides of the tray, and incorporate bilateral stimulation. I will be using these little gadgets, pulsars," I said.

I reached down to the floor and picked up a container, grabbed the pulsars, and showed them to Jane. The pulsars are approximately two inches in size, battery operated, placed in the palm of each hand of the client, and when turned on give a light vibration. The sensation of this is not painful, and many of my clients tell me it is relaxing. Jane said her former EMDR therapist used a lightbar, which is a visual form of bilateral stimulation. I prefer using the pulsars when I am combining EMDR with IFSsandtray because the client is looking at the figures in the tray, not a lightbar.

"Jane, this is one way I work when someone has two Parts with opposing viewpoints," I said. "When we go into the sandplay room I will ask you to pick out two miniatures. You will place one figure that represents the Part that is shameful on one side, then place the Part that knows it didn't do anything wrong on the other side of the tray, and I will talk directly to both. Most likely these two Parts are Protectors, have the same positive intention for you, and both have their own unique ways of trying to help. Often neither one understands the other—they are divided—yet both want the same outcome for you: to be safe and not triggered by the wounded exile who holds the original wound in your system."

I asked Jane if she understood what was happening with her Parts. She told me she did, and we went into the sandplay room. Once inside, I asked her to find the miniature that best represented her feeling shameful. She walked around the room, looked at many of the human figurines, and stopped in front of the sexual miniatures. She stood there for a few minutes, and I waited without saying a word. She picked a figure and said, "I have no idea why I picked this one." She opened her hand and showed me the miniature before she placed it into the tray. It was a small carved wooden smoking pipe shaped in the form of a woman that I purchased in Key West at a smoke shop. This woman was naked and had her legs spread wide open, exposing her vulva. Her left hand covered her eyes, and her right hand held the inside of her right knee (Figure 13.1).

I asked Jane to place the miniature either on the right or left side of the tray, place it close to the side, and in the middle. I then asked her to find the miniature that felt she didn't do anything wrong. Jane once again got up and moved about the room (Figure 13.2). She came back with the same leather-clad miniature she used in Chapter 12. At that time the figurine wanted to be

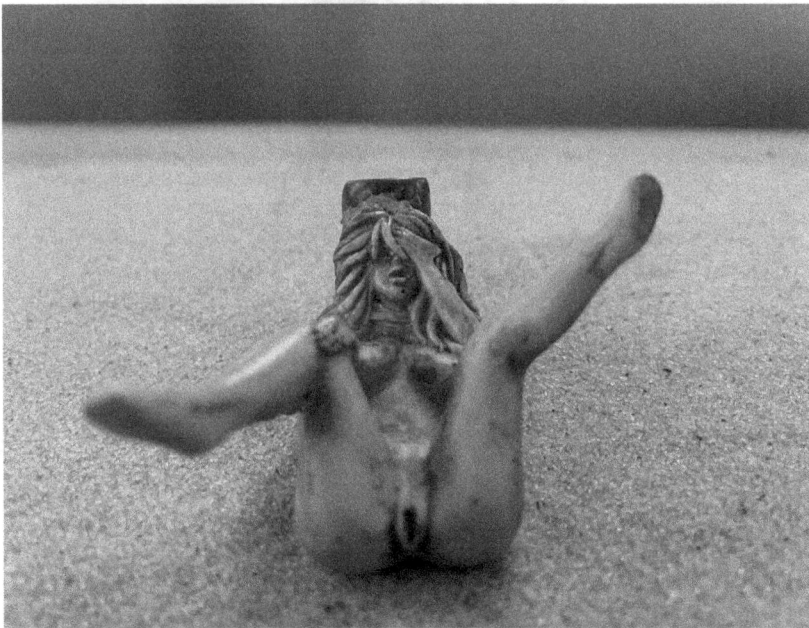

Figure 13.1 Shameful

Photo by the author

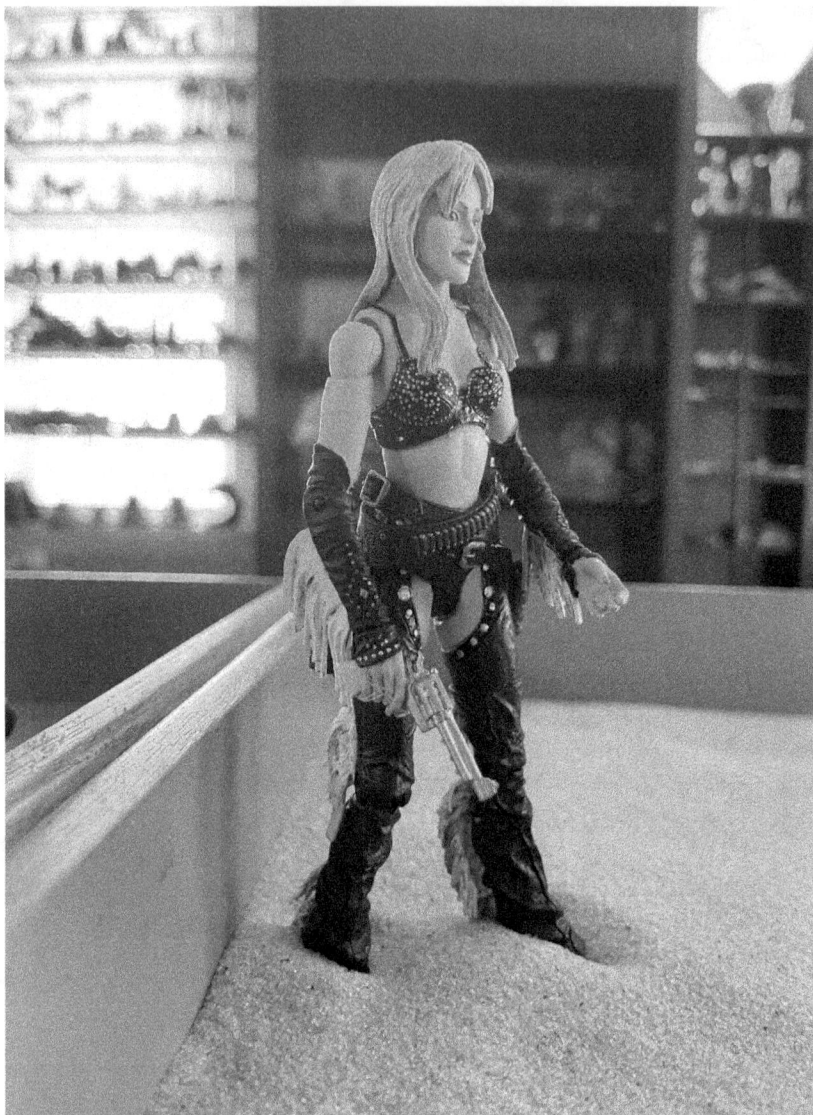

Figure 13.2 Part That Didn't Feel It Did Anything Wrong

Photo by the author

known by the name, Bitch (see Chapter 12, "Jane: Letting Go of Painful Sex Through IFSsandtray").

"Jane, place this figure that represents the Part of you that says, 'I didn't do anything wrong' in the tray on the left side in the middle

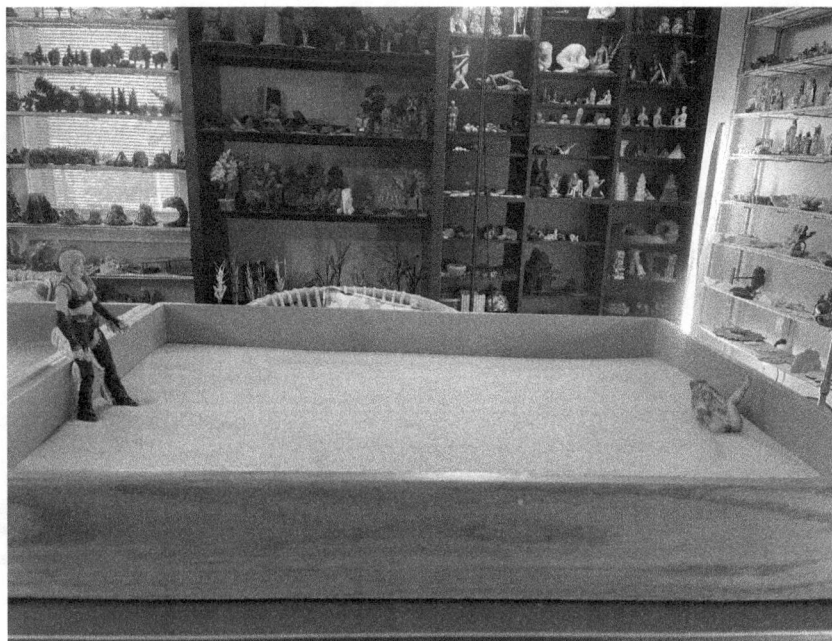

Figure 13.3 Polarized Parts

Photo by the author

opposite of the one that is shameful," I said, watching Jane place it into the tray (Figure 13.3).

Jane then sat down. I had already placed the pulsars under the steel cart holding the tray while she was picking the two miniatures so she could have easy access to them.

"Jane, pick up the pulsars underneath the table, place one in each hand, and let's check what speed feels right for you. I am going to turn them on and you're not going to have to do anything except tell me what speed feels right. You will know when it feels right." I watched while she settled. "Okay let me know when we have the exact right speed."

I turned the pulsars on and watched Jane's face and body. I slowed them down and Jane said it was too slow. I turned it up, and she said it was too fast. Finally, we found exactly the right speed, and we settled in for the processing of her two polarized Parts.

"Jane," I said, "now I am going to put the pulsars on and keep them on throughout, if you decide you want to stop just say so or if you feel you can't say anything just raise your hand so I will know to turn them off."

If you, the reader, are an EMDR therapist, I know this is not how you have been trained to use EMDR. I had been certified in EMDR for many years before I began to utilize or combine it with my work with IFSsandtray. I've discovered my clients often find the pulsars helpful when we are processing sandtray work. However, I never apply any form of bilateral stimulation when I do a Kalffian sandplay session; they are very different modalities (see Chapter 3, "What Path to Choose: The Difference: Sandtray or Sandplay"). The reason I never utilize EMDR in Kalffian Sandplay is that modality is structured and all clinicians who utilized Kalffian sandplay follow the same process, unlike the modality of Sandtray. No outside influences are needed or necessary and would alter the sandplay process as it was intended.

"Jane, what I want you to do is look at the miniature that represents shame, and tell me why you picked this miniature?"

"I picked it because it's sexual, it's vulnerable," she said before pausing for 5 seconds and adding, "she *feels* conflicted."

I repeated Jane's words, "*She feels conflicted.*" I paused before adding, "Jane, can you tell me about *how* she feels conflicted? She represents the Part of you that felt shame on Sunday when your son came home earlier than you expected. Just focus on that feeling *she* is having now." I paused for a few moments to give Jane time to focus on the shameful Part in front of her.

"I can sense you are feeling it now in your body. I am witnessing you move in the chair. How do you notice it showing up in your body?"

"I feel nausea and my lower back hurts." Jane paused, then she pointed to her chest, "I feel it here too."

I validated her immediately by responding, "Yes. I can see that." I paused and then added, "I can also hear how much you are sensing her in your body. I am going to ask you to do something. Focus on the figurine, you see her in front of you on the right side of the tray and you feel something in your chest, lower back, and in your stomach like nausea. Just notice those sensations. Focus on her while you focus on your body sensations in your chest, lower back, and stomach. Can you describe the chest pain?"

Jane physically moved in her chair, leaned forward, and then bent over. She made a moaning sound, and I witnessed her physically changing in front of me. Jane was feeling in her body what the Part was experiencing in its body. I see this all the time when I am working with clients and their Parts.

"Augh!" she groaned.

"I hear it's really hard." I paused and then whispered: "I see you hunched over." I also copied her vocalization of the "augh sound," repeating it back to her in the same tone.

She replied, "I really feel nausea in the stomach."

At this point in the session, I switched into a more hypnotic style of language. I kept my voice soft and modulated, sustaining a gentle cadence. I wanted her to concentrate on her body. I was observing her breathe in and out. On each exhale I would say to her "That's right," or something similar, or I'd just pause. When she inhaled, I would direct her to focus internally again. I represent that below, with three dots (...) in the dialogue that follows.

"Yes. So can you now focus on the sensations happening in your chest, lower back, and the nausea in your stomach, all at once ... Focus on all three sensations at the same time ... If you want to close your eyes, you can, so you can really focus internally ... you can focus internally and notice all the sensations happening at the same time ... Notice them now ... Focus on when you felt all three sensations in the same identical way you have felt the pain in your chest ... lower back ... and nausea ... in the same exact way before in your life ... and where does that take you ... Do you have a memory, or a scene that comes to mind?" I paused again.

"Ahhh, third grade. Maybe fourth grade," she said. "Yeah, fourth grade I was doing a project in school, and I thought we were screwing it up. We were making brownies!" She said in a raised voice, and I saw her face. It appeared she couldn't believe it. "And I just felt like the world was going to end if screwed it up, I felt horrible, and less than."

"Yes ... I want you to focus on being in that fourth grade experience, now ... making the brownies ... focus on making the brownies ... as if you were there now ... now is then and then is now ... focus on making those brownies as if you are in the fourth grade now ... feel the feelings and see if there's something else that goes on in your chest, in your back, and notice the nausea happening in your stomach ... see if there is another sensation or another feeling of what's going on there ... as you focus on your back, chest, and nausea ... as if you're in fourth grade now ... as you are there now ... be there now as if you are in the fourth grade making those brownies ... is there another—"

I was just about to finish the question, Jane interjected. "There's massive fear."

I have been trained in hypnosis, and in that moment, I knew she was in a hypnotic state. "Yes, fear. I get that." I said, talking gently to that Part of her that was feeling shame.

"Fear and I am just so fearful."

"Fearful ... focus on that fearful feeling in fourth grade ... where do you feel the fear in your body in the fourth grade?" I asked.

"I feel the hair on my arms standing up."

I looked at her arms and noticed they were moving slightly.

"Yes, focus on the hair on your arms standing up ... and imagine being in fourth grade now ... as you are there now ... now is then and then is now ... focus on the hair standing up on your arms with the fearful feeling ... when you felt the sensation of the hair standing up on your arms in exactly in the same way when you were in fourth grade ... where does that take you?... to a scene or an age when you felt the hair standing up and nausea in your stomach before fourth grade."

Jane responded immediately with, "When my mom dropped me off at our church for my weekly religious education. She left me there, and we didn't have any classes .... There was this guy. He was a teacher who wanted me to get into his car and I said, 'No. No. I can't get into your car!'"

"Yeah. Focus on when he wanted you to get into his car ... focus on that now as the guy wanted you to get into the car ... be there now ... when he asked you to get in his car ... focus on that and how you didn't want to get into the car, and you didn't do it ..." I said, my voice still modulated.

Jane didn't take more than three seconds to respond, "I have an abandoned feeling and I feel nausea. I am scared, and shameful because I said no, I feel bad for saying no to the guy. There's shame there and I am just really scared."

"Focus on that shame because you said no to the guy ... the shame of saying no to the guy ... focus how you feel fearful, nausea, and shame because you said no ... focus on all of that at the same time ... that feeling of saying no combined with the shame ... just focus ... what's happening now as you are there at that moment?"

"I am walking and he's following me. I am going over to the church so I can call somebody." Jane's voice became softer, quieter, and her face looked as if she was scared. The sides of her mouth went down and she physically swallowed. "I am feeling shameful because I have a new hat on and it's snowing. I don't want to ruin the hat because my parents will get mad at me."

"Now, focus on walking and you're afraid of ruining the hat ... focus on the feeling of walking and not wanting your parents getting mad at you .... focus on what you feel when you're possibly going to ruin the hat and you don't want your parents to get angry now ... what's happening in your body as you're walking over to use the phone at the church now?"

"It feels like my body is crumbling in" she said without a moment's hesitation.

"Yes. Focus on that crumbling in, just focus on the crumbling feeling now ... focus on how the body of crumbling in feels."

"Same, same, it's crumbling in. Just getting the nausea, the fear on my arms, and chest. Just feeling it all."

"Yes, that's right," I said. "Just focus on all those feelings and sensations in your body together … just notice all your body sensations … when you felt those same sensations in the exact same way when you were younger than being dropped off at the church."

"When I was younger, I don't know, maybe kindergarten. I am running into the middle of the road in front of a car that's coming down the street. I am upset because my dad is screaming at me. I feel so much shame."

"When your dad screamed at you for running down the middle of the road and you feel shame … focus on him screaming at you now, as if then is now and now is then … focus on your body as you are running down the middle of the road."

"There's another Part of me there now," she said, shifting in her seat. "It's saying, 'why aren't you people taking care of me?'"

"Yeah, ask that Part that just asked why people aren't taking care of you, to step back … now, focus on the body when your dad is screaming, and you feel the shame … sense how your body feels the sensations in that moment as if the moment is happening now … just focus on that shame, that fear, and dad yelling at you … sense if you had those same exact feelings before kindergarten … focus on the nausea in your body … anything come earlier"

"Yeah, there's another time when I was in kindergarten. I did something wrong, and I had to stay in during recess. I was just beside myself. I felt shame … my dad is going to yell at me," she said, again shifting into the present tense.

"As you are staying in for recess … and you did something wrong … focus on being beside yourself …. focus on your body as you felt shame … and dad is going to yell at you" I said.

"I feel like I am a bad person. So, all these things there's an underlying theme."

"Okay, don't analyze … just go with the feelings in the body, now," I said gently.

"So, the feeling is you're bad."

"Focus on your bad … your dad screaming … on those sensations in your body …. focus on your dad screaming … your fear of your dad yelling at you …. when did you feel the same fear … I am bad … and notice your body … and when did you feel the same sensations in your body?"

"I remember being in the backyard and I had a bathing suit on, and the strap fell off my shoulder. And we were throwing water balloons at each other having fun and he wasn't mad at me. Then he became angry and began yelling at me for no reason. I felt ashamed and I was a bad person again."

"Focus on when you're throwing water at your dad ... just notice how your dad is yelling ... he's screaming ... just let your mind go to the first time he yelled at you ... focus on the first time he ever possibly yelled at you ... what do you get?"

She shook her head. "Can't get it."

"All right, okay ... we're going to start with the time in your backyard when you're throwing water ... focus on the water .... I wonder if you see the little girl who is being yelled at by her dad?"

"Hmm hump," she said, nodding her head. "I see her." "As you see her. How do you feel towards her?"

Jane paused for five seconds. "Compassionate," she said.

I was thrilled because I was hoping she would say one of the eight 'C' words, confidence, calmness, creativity, clarity, curiosity, courage, compassion, and connectedness used in the IFS model. I now knew Jane was able to start the healing process for herself and all the little ones we had just met. She was experiencing Self energy and ready to proceed. We had reached the beginning of where she was shamed.

"Yes, can you send her compassion. Can you do that?" I asked

"Yes. I can."

"As you see her. See if you can be in the scene with her as your adult Self?"

"Yes, I am there with her now."

"Where is she and where are you?"

"She is up the stairs."

"Ask her to see or sense you."

"She senses me," she said.

"Yes, as she senses you ask her if she knows who you are."

"Yes! She does know me!" Jane said in a surprised voice. I smiled even though she couldn't see me. I was so happy for her at this point. She was on her way of healing herself from this terrible experience that left her feeling full of shame.

"Ask her if she trusts you?"

"Yes. She trusts me."

"Ask her to tell you more about all of her pain and shame. About the scene with dad. Let her show you all her pain. And you as an adult just witness it."

Jane was silent for approximately ninety seconds. "Okay. She showed me."

At this point I followed what I learned in my IFS training to heal that exile. I worked with Jane to heal that little girl who carried all that shame from when her father got angry. Now, as I guided Jane through this, that little girl left the scene with her dad with confidence. She wanted to leave the yard and was now walking in the woods with Jane. This little girl was now healed and no longer carried shame in her young body.

We then did the same process with the little girl whose bathing suit strap fell down. She, too, healed like the little girl. Next, we addressed the Part that felt like she was bad when Dad was screaming. She healed also. Then the Part of Jane that ran into the middle of the road also healed. Then we healed the Part that was dropped off at CCD (religious education school), followed by the fourth grader who was baking the brownies. After all these exiles were healed, we turned back to the recent episode when her son walked into the house. Jane was able to feel differently about that experience that occurred three days earlier. I asked Jane how she felt now about what happened.

She replied, "I feel like I have more compassion for myself, and kids walk in on their friggin' parents all the time. I know he didn't hear us."

"Fabulous. Now I want you to find the miniature that represents the new felt sense of that shameful part now with confidence."

Jane got up and selected an angel with open arms and she said (Figure 13.4), "This is how I feel now. 'I am free.' This angel represents hope, vulnerability, and kindness to me. She is strong."

I looked at it, smiled, and realized the open legs were now replaced with open arms! Then asked her to find the miniature that started with the belief, "I didn't do anything wrong. She now wants to be called, 'I am free'."

She got up, found another miniature, and replaced the figure that once represented Bitch. The new figure was a woman dressed in a white tank top, jeans, and shoulder-length blonde hair.

This figure seemed more like Jane. Maybe on the weekends. [see photo below] After she placed this figure in the tray I asked, "What's her name?"

Jane said without hesitation, "This is Belinda." She knows she didn't do anything wrong. Maybe she's a revision of Bitch."

"Well, let's wait and see about that. We will have to see if Bitch shows up again. Then we will know. For now, let's celebrate Belinda!" I said (Figure 13.5).

"Okay, Jane, one last thing. When 'I am free,' and Belinda are working together, find the miniature that best represents how they work together."

Jane once again went to look for just the right miniature. She looked for about thirty seconds, came back to the tray, and placed a nude couple into the center of the tray.

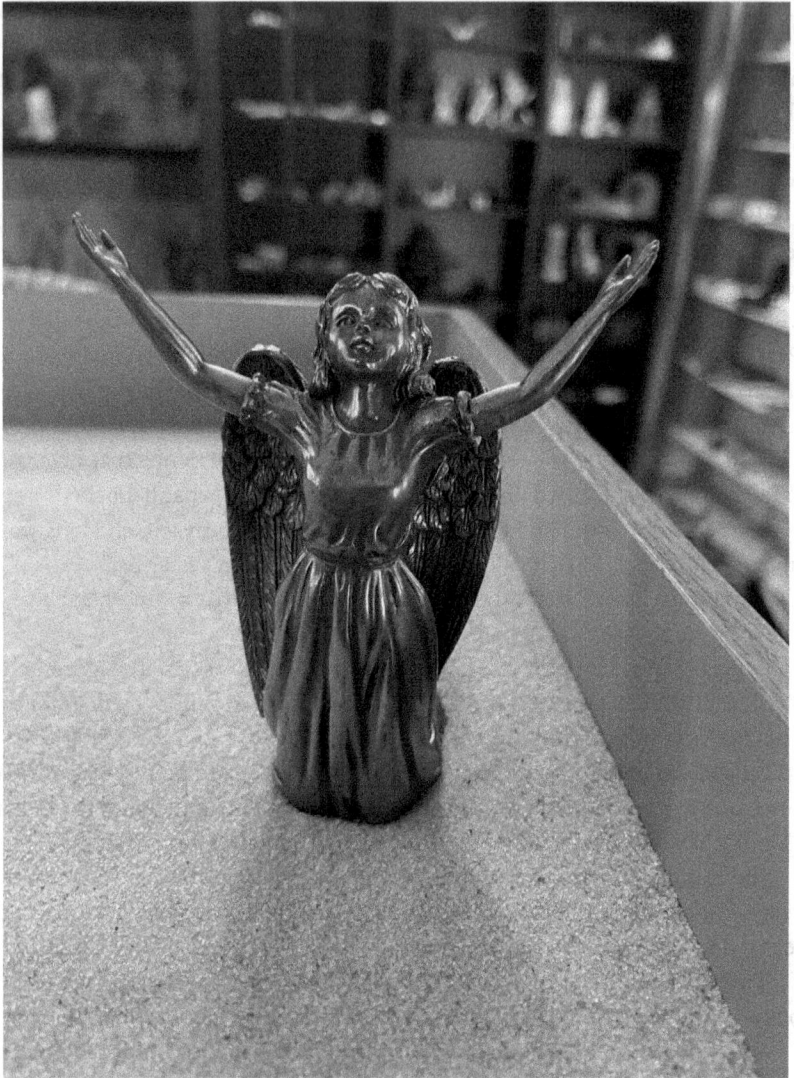

Figure 13.4 I Am Free

Photo by the author

"This is me and David." she said (Figure 13.6).

I recognized immediately the freedom she now expressed. After the incident with her son that elicited so much shame, she had chosen a figure that was vulnerable, open, yet trying to hide. With the angel representing freedom, and Belinda representing a composed, relaxed state, she was

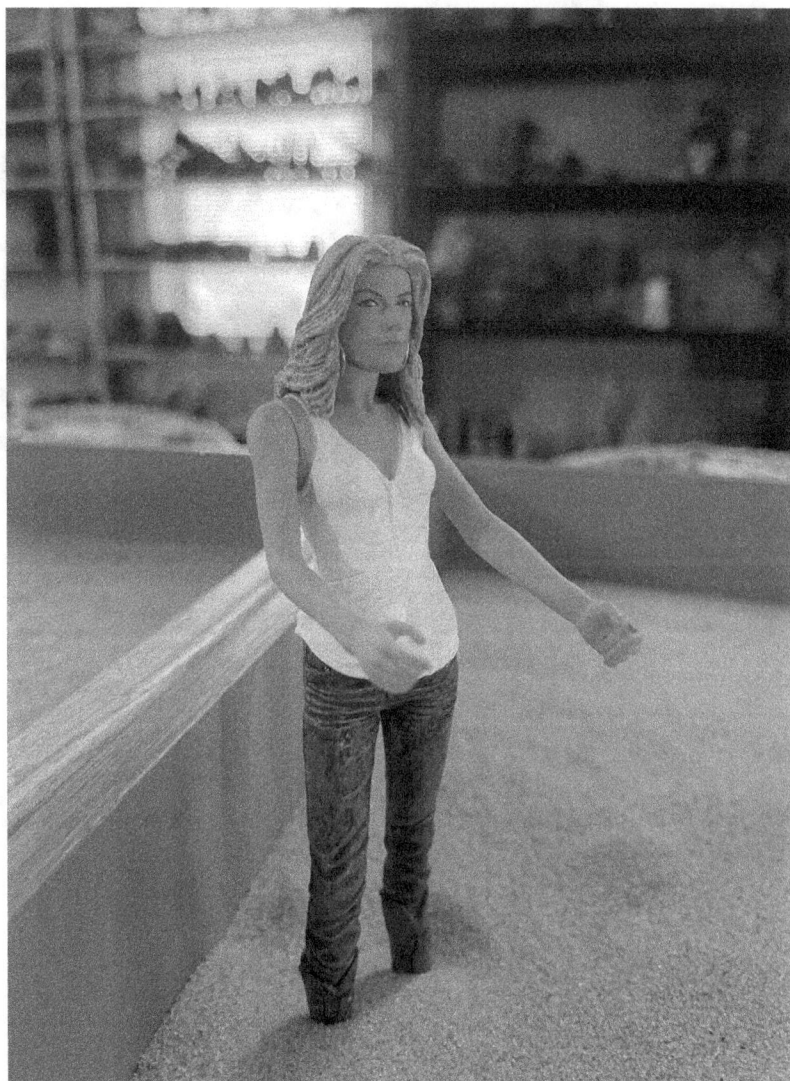

Figure 13.5 Belinda

Photo by the author

integrating the two main Parts that were polarized. By acknowledging how her Parts could now work together, she could find pleasure and freedom in her lovemaking.

Jane and I continued to work together for eight more months. She healed the Parts that she once hated and realized how they did help her. I will never

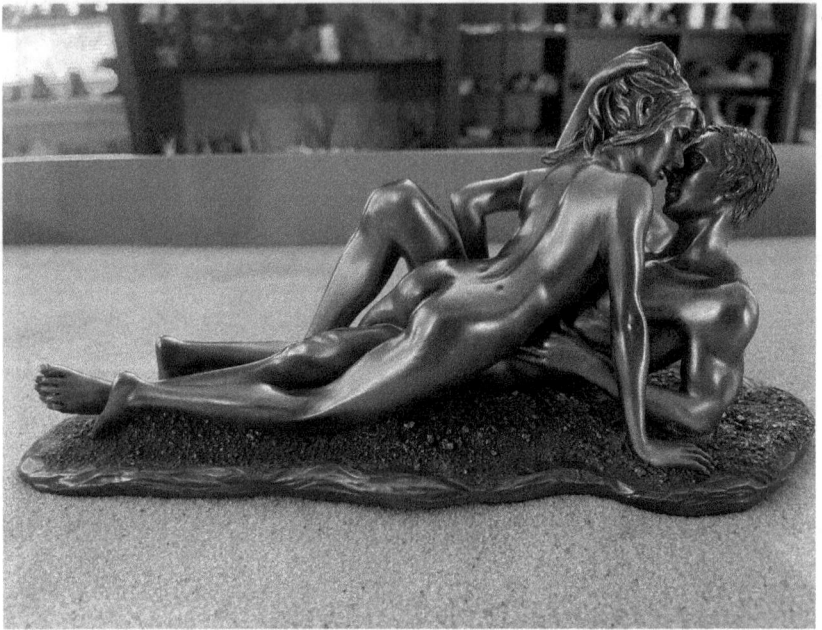

Figure 13.6 Jane and David

Photo by the author

forget the day we said our goodbyes. First, she called Harvey, my therapy dog, over to her side and hugged him, kissed the top of his forehead, and said, "Harvey, you are a special boy."

I had a tear in my eye when she looked up at me and asked if we could also hug. I said, "Of course."

We embraced and she then whispered, "I can't thank you enough for how you helped me. I never thought I would be ever to have sex again. This type of therapy changed me forever."

"Jane, I couldn't have done it without you."

Section Three
Clinical Exercises

Internal Family Systems Directives to Use with Clients

14

> Remember, what happens in that inner world has tremendous implications for what happens in the outside world.
>
> (Dr. Richard Schwartz)

This chapter introduces two IFSsandtray directives to use with clients, one with the option to utilize Eye Movement Desensitization Reprocessing (EMDR) pulsers and the other without. Both of these instructions are highly influenced by Internal Family Systems (IFS) which has been adapted to using a sand tray and miniature figurines. Externalizing Parts in a sand tray allows both clinician and client to clearly see representations of the client's Parts as miniature figurines and makes following the client's therapeutic process easier,

Betty, the client, was ecstatic about the work she was doing and found it more helpful than talk therapy, which she had been doing for 15 years with other therapists. Please note, she signed a release for the pictures you are about to see.

The first IFSsandtray discussed below introduces the reader to the best way to prepare for a session combining IFS and The Polyvagal Theory while utilizing sand and miniatures. This first directive and technique is called, "IFS / PVT IFSsandtray." Directions and sand tray photos below will illustrate major IFS constructs of how each emotion is called a Part (see Chapter 5, "Multiplicity: Introduction to Parts in Therapy"). In addition, by utilizing miniatures this allows the client to externalize Parts. At the same time introduces the client to the states of the autonomic nervous system.

DOI: 10.4324/9781003388302-17

Experiential Exercise: IFS/PVT IFSsandtray Part One

To start the first part of this IFS/PVT IFSsandtray experiential are listed below in sequential order.

Clinician must understand concepts of IFS and PVT.

1. Allocate one full session consisting of 45–50 minutes for this exercise.
2. If possible, use two trays. If the clinician doesn't own any sand trays, use a section of the floor or any flat surface approximately 20-by-30 inches. Later in the process, the client will be moving the miniatures into another space, a similar size area would be advised. Creativity in the clinician is a bonus.
3. Have figures or objects which are listed below and have four small containers available which can hold three to five miniatures each. This will be helpful for the client to separate figurines that are going to represent four of their emotional states.
4. Essential miniatures to make available for clients:
   a. Objects displaying qualities, such as calmness, playfulness, happiness, etc.
   b. Objects exhibiting productiveness, achievements, proactivity, gardening, dancing, celebrating, etc.
   c. Objects representing anger, frustration, jealousy, reactivity, and substances, such as alcohol, drugs, or cigarettes, etc.
   d. Objects showing how it might look if one feels hopelessness, helplessness, or giving up, examples include a bed, sad figures, etc.
5. Clinician should give the client an explanation of what they are about to do with sand and miniatures. Simplifying language is helpful for many clients who haven't been introduced to the IFS concept of emotions labeled as Parts or the different states of PVT.
6. During this explanation the clinician should reassure the client the exercise is designed to allow ease in comprehending these unfamiliar concepts.
   a. Example: the clinician might say, "The figurines you are going to select are representations of basic emotions all humans have."
      i. "You will pick three or four miniatures which represent when you feel calm, happy, confident, or in a Zen-like state."
      ii. "The next set will be when you are managing things in your life or doing a job with ease and being proactive."
      iii. "The third set are emotions such as anger, rage, feeling walled off, being reactive etc."

      iv.   "Finally, the last group will be when you are feeling like giving up, collapsed, helpless, hopeless, shameful, or guilty, etc."

      v.   "You will label each aspect of the exercise with the word that fits for you, we will be going over this in our work together going forward. If you don't want to place your hands in the sand don't. Most importantly have fun learning these new concepts."

7. Give the four containers to the client and suggest they go to the miniatures and place each set of figurines in separate containers. Once the client has picked all the miniatures go to the sand tray.

8. The clinician will ask their client to put the first set of miniatures, which represent feeling calm, calm, happy, confident, or in a Zen-like state into the sand tray.

    a.   Ask them to place these miniatures one by one closest to the wall in a horizontal line.

    b.   Invite the client to tell you what each figure represents to themselves as they place it in the row.

    c.   After the client has placed all three or four miniatures in the row, the clinician asks the client to name that row in their own words.

9. With enthusiasm, the clinician will repeat what the client called the row of miniatures and add, "this also known as Self in Internal Family Systems and ventral vagal in The Polyvagal Theory."

    a.   For example, after the client places and describes each miniature in the row, the clinician repeats back while pointing to, but not touching the miniatures, "That is a great representation of your happy place (if that is the words the client uses to describe the Self or ventral vagal state), in Internal Family Systems or IFS for short this is called Self and in the Polyvagal Theory this is called the ventral vagal state. We will discuss more of these concepts in-depth during our future sessions."

10. Clinicians should inquire how the client may feel both emotionally and describe any physical sensations there may be in their body when they are in this state.

    a.   Body sensations are important as sensations can be associated with somatic reactions from Parts.

    b.   The client may experience these sensations without conscious awareness.

    c.   The clinician should pause, let the individual connect with the sensations in their body consciously which will help them in their therapy going forward.

11. Finish this row. Next the clinician will smooth out the sand with a brush or their palm which will remove any marks in the sand from where the miniatures were placed and move to the next container which will become the second row. This will be with the manager Parts or in the proactive behavior which is one way the autonomic nervous system (ANS) mobilizes.
12. Repeat 9–11.
13. Finish row two and go to the third row. This will be with the firefighter Parts, or reactive behavior, which is another way the ANS system mobilizes.
14. Repeat 9–11.
15. Finish row three and go to the fourth row. This will be the exiled Parts, or collapsed behavior, which is another way the ANS immobilizes, called dorsal vagal in PVT.

The following images, 14.1 through 14.5, are based on an earlier IFS/ PVT IFSsandtray with Betty. During that session, she was able to comprehend how her autonomic nervous system was directly related to her Parts and behaviors.

Betty's personality reflected a loving, selfless, friendly, and approachable individual. She selected four miniatures to represent Self in IFS or Ventral vagal in The Polyvagal Theory. In the first row, she placed an angel with praying hands with a heart by its feet. The second item was a rock. Both of these had the word love written on them. Two others, one a silver smiling, upright human figure with outstretched arms, palms facing up, and a character from the movie *Monsters, Inc.* grinning and raising its left arm, possibly saying "hi." These images did align with qualities seen in Betty's outgoing temperament. See Figure 14.1.

When Betty selected her objects exhibiting productiveness, achievements, proactivity, and celebration, she chose a house, a lotus, and a fairy holding something in her left hand. Betty explained why she selected these miniatures, saying the house represented how she liked to clean around the house, take care of household chores, and pay bills. The lotus reminded her of gardening which she loved to do. The fairy with the staff reminded her she could do everything and get everything done. She ultimately called this row her "getting things done" state (see Figure 14.2).

Betty next selected figurines representing her anger, frustration, being walled off, and reactivity. First, she chose the angry figure from the movie "Inside Out." This miniature had flames coming out of its head, an angry face gritting its teeth, and its left hand raised in a fist. The second figurine was

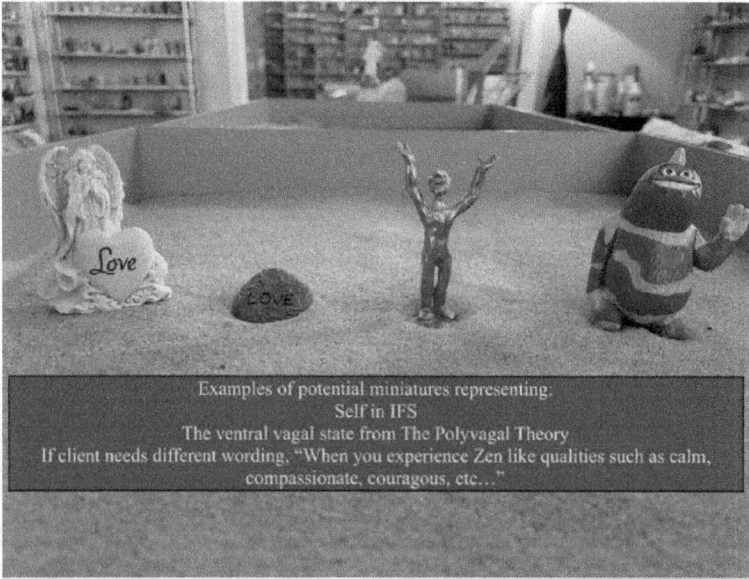

Figure 14.1 Examples of Potential Self Miniatures

Photo by the author

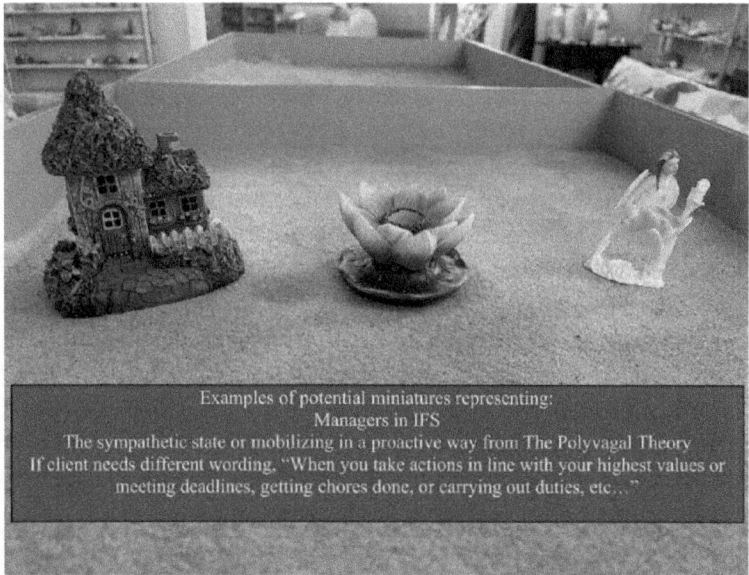

Figure 14.2 Examples of Potential Miniatures Representing Managers in IFS

Photo by the author

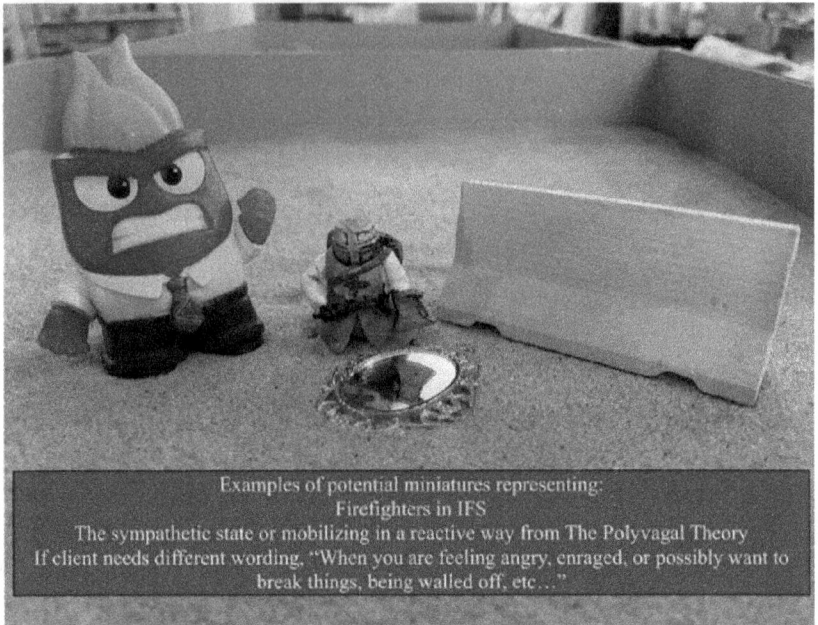

Examples of potential miniatures representing:
Firefighters in IFS
The sympathetic state or mobilizing in a reactive way from The Polyvagal Theory
If client needs different wording, "When you are feeling angry, enraged, or possibly want to break things, being walled off, etc…"

Figure 14.3 Examples of Potential Miniatures Representing Firefighters in IFS
Photo by the author

smaller, with a flattened head wrapped in armor, holding an axe., Just below the axe Betty placed a mirror while saying, "when I get angry, I just want to break things!" The last figure in this row was a miniature concrete construction barrier found in street detours. Betty said, "this is when I feel walled off from everyone?" She called this row her angry state (see Figure 14.3).

When Betty selected the objects showing how she experienced hopelessness, helplessness, and giving up, she put in the tray a four-poster bed with a purple and yellow flower mattress and pillow, a gray-colored faceless figure lying on top of the mattress, its hands up to where its mouth would be, a yellow patchworked miniature quilt covering the miniature figure. Beside this, she placed a yellow non-binary figure with its head in the sand, and a white plastic figure of a woman with a ponytail holding her stomach with her left arm, and the other arm holding up her downward-facing head. Betty called this her sad and depressed state (see Figure 14.4).

Once all figurines were placed in the tray it will look like the picture below, showing a bird's eye view of this portion of the session (see Figure 14.5).

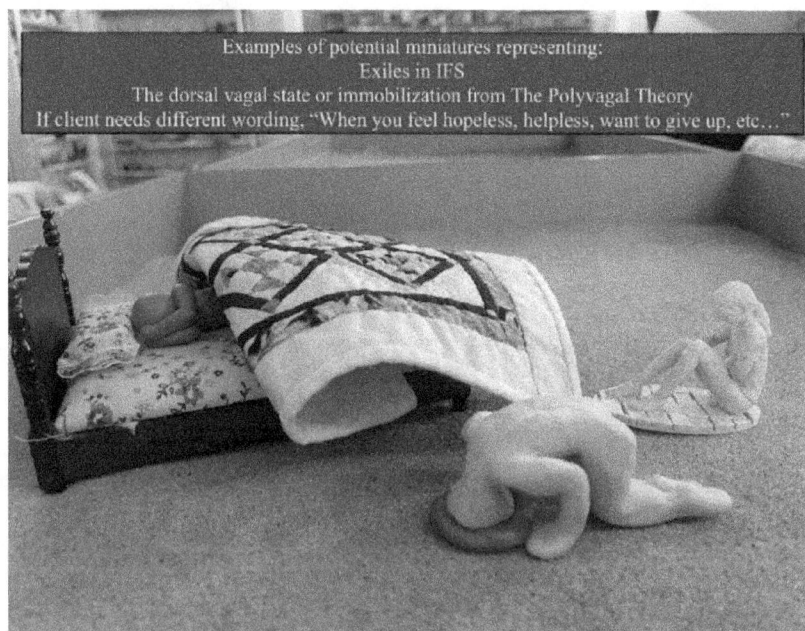

Figure 14.4 Examples of Potential Miniatures Representing Exiles in IFS

Photo by the author

Experiential Exercise: IFS/PVT IFSsandtray Part Two

The second part of this exercise is significant because the client has just ended up feeling like they are in a dorsal vagal state where their body can experience sensations of hopelessness. The miniatures representing Parts in the dorsal or exiled state are collapsed, helpless, and hopeless—exactly where the exiled Part was trapped in time. They may be experiencing some of these feelings in a profound manner because they have become aligned with the miniatures.

When the client is engaging in this exercise their autonomic nervous system (ANS) mobilizes as if the individual had moved the dorsal vagal state. The Parts, body, and mind don't know if what just happened was real or not, they all react as if they just experienced the immobilized state.

It's important to take the client back into the ventral or Self-state where they first started before they leave the session. It is important to be aware of the time left in the session.

1. Clinician asks the client to take one of the figures in the fourth row which represents their sadness, hopelessness, or helplessness and place

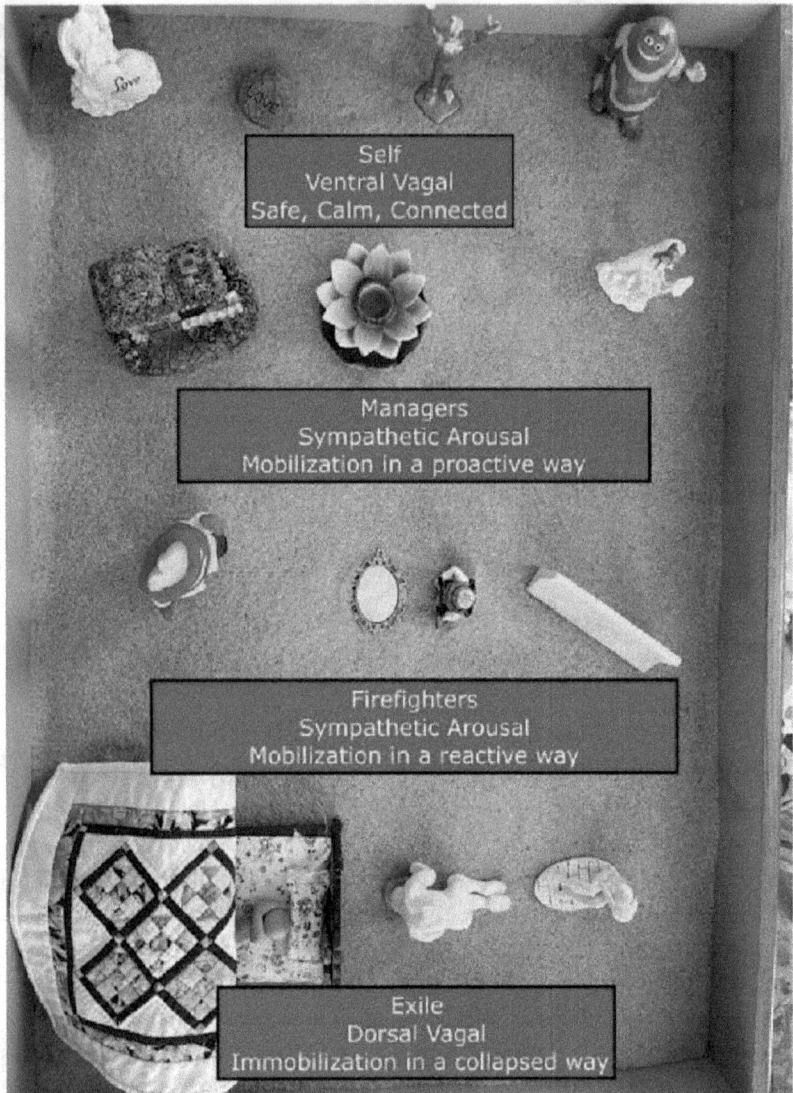

Figure 14.5 Top View of Miniatures Representing Both IFS and Polyvagal Theory
Photo by the author

that miniature in the second sand tray. (For Betty it was the hopelessness Part shown as the figure with its head in the sand. See Figure 14.6). Alternatively, they can place the figure in the cleared location if the clinician doesn't have a second tray.

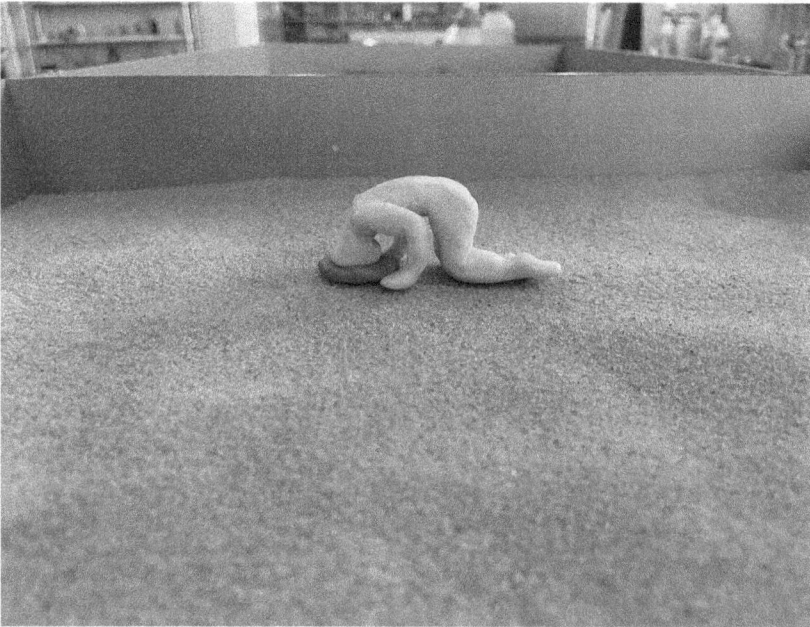

Figure 14.6 Head in the Sand

Photo by the author

2. The clinician asks the client what that figure needs to do to move out of this state, and if there are any figures which could help this, Part. (For Betty it was going to bed to sleep, see Figure 14.7.)

3. The clinician asks the client what could they do to help these Parts or miniatures help them move or mobilize themselves out of that state? Clients will most likely select a figure from their proactive or managers in the second row. If they don't, ask them to find another miniature that would be able to help at that moment.

   • Betty said she could repeat the serenity prayer and began to say it at that moment. With this, her body began mobilizing in the chair, and she waved her arms. This, she said, gives her hope, peacefulness, and she was no longer feeling as sad. She added the house and lotus from the proactive or manager section of the tray alongside the head-in-the-sand figure and the bed. She discussed how she loved gardening, which brought her peace of mind, calmed her down, and helped her feel great. This is mobilization in a proactive way (see Figure 14.8).

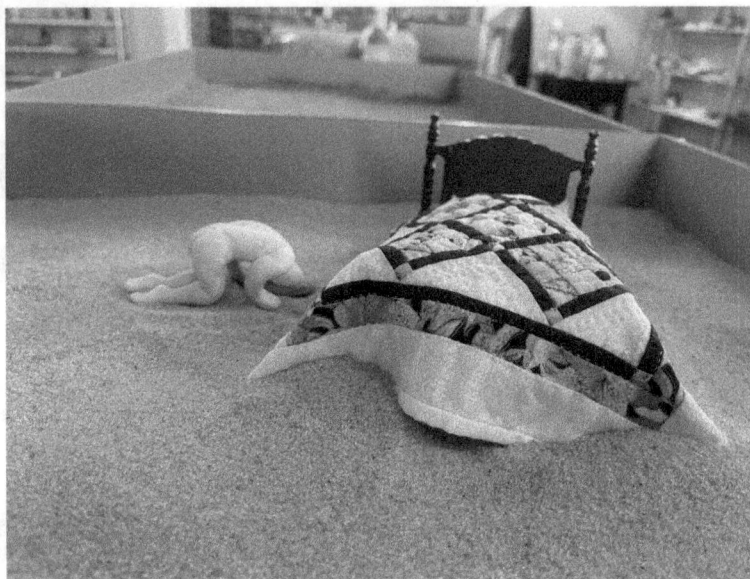

Figure 14.7 Head in the Sand and Bed with Handmade Quilt

Photo by the author

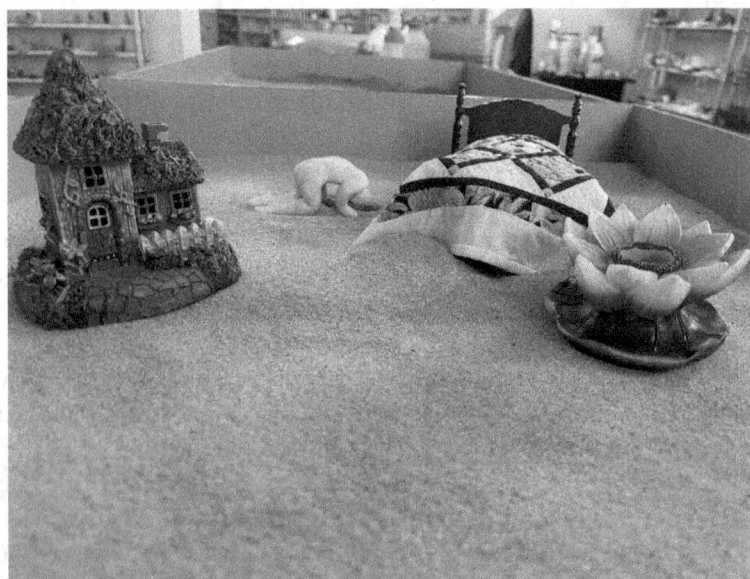

Figure 14.8 Mobilization in a Proactive Way

Photo by the author

4. The clinician asks the client what happens next? This is when the client will most likely use the miniatures that they used for Self, which are typically the ones selected to represent calm, happiness, confidence, or in a Zen-like state.

   • Betty moved the happy figure, the rock with the word love on it, and the silver figure with its arms and hands in the air. She discussed how happy she felt, felt the love she had for others, and the love others had for her after she says the serenity prayer. The result was her ability to get out of bed. This brought her into the ventral vagal state (see Figure 14.9).

5. The clinician then recaps what just happened in the IFS/PVT IFSsandtray session they just completed together.

The clinician will discuss how the client moved out of the dorsal vagal, through sympathetic arousal, and back into the ventral vagal or Self state with the individual. The sand tray, which is now in front of them, displays how that process was completed. Clients often enjoy the recap as they are have come to a better understanding of IFS and PVT.

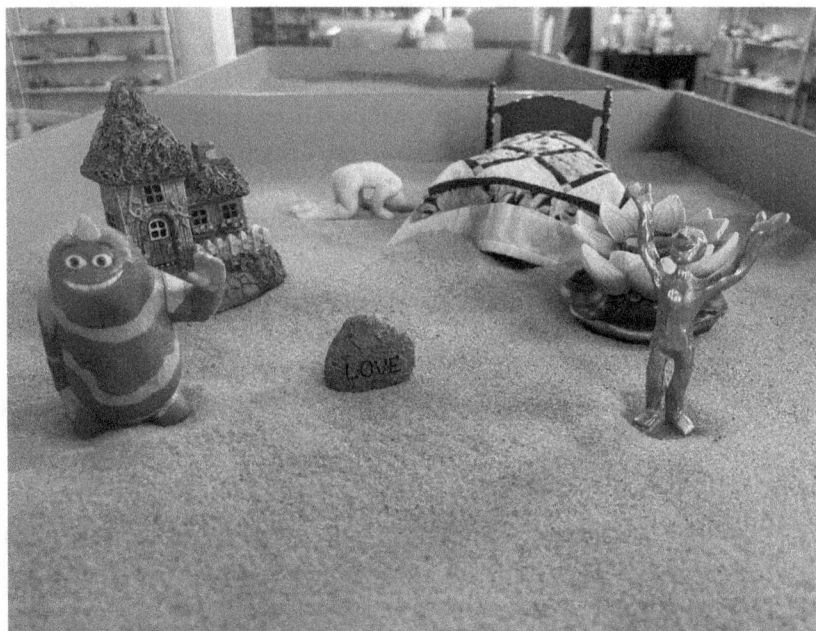

Figure 14.9 Self Images

Photo by the author

Experiential Exercise: IFS/Zen/EMDR IFSsandtray

The second directive displays another IFSsandtray technique called, "IFS/Zen/EMDR IFSsandtray." Two sand trays are utilized, one will hold miniatures representing a Zen-like state or Self in IFS. The other will be the working tray, which will be set up with the presenting problem. Clinician should be in their own Zen state and allow themselves to be spontaneous, flexible, and open to their own creativity when doing this experiential exercise. This will be different every time as each client has various presenting problems.

IFS/Zen/EMDR IFSsandtray experiential are also listed below in sequential order:

1. Allocate approximately 35–40 minutes for this experiential exercise.
2. Notice time throughout the session and tell the client that you will let them know when there are approximately ten minutes left.
   a. Reassure the client a lot can be achieved in 35–40 minutes.
3. Provide two containers for the client to put their miniatures in.
4. Ask the client what issue they would like to work on in that session.
5. Repeat the problem back to the client and ask them if you understood the presenting issue.
   a. The presenting issue Betty wanted to work on was to have a voice and be able to discuss her dissatisfaction with her boyfriend's point of view. He wanted to have family dinners with her and her two young adult grandchildren.
   b. The grandchildren were both in their early twenties.
6. Ask the client to pick four to six miniatures, which represent themselves when they are in a Zen-like state or feeling calm, curious, connected, and compassionate. Place those miniatures in one of the containers.
7. Once those miniatures have been selected ask the client to pick another few figurines to represent the presenting problem, one they would like to have more clarity about.
   a. Betty selected some of the figures directly from her IFS/PVT IFSsandtray.
   b. She brought back her bed as she could rest and relax there,
8. When the client sits in front of the sand trays, ask them to place their Zen-like figures in a row facing the other tray. Have them tell you what each of these miniatures means and how it helps them. See Figure 14.10.

   Have the client make a scene of the problem in the other tray. Ask the client to explain these individual miniatures as they place them in the tray in a way it makes sense. See Figure 14.11.

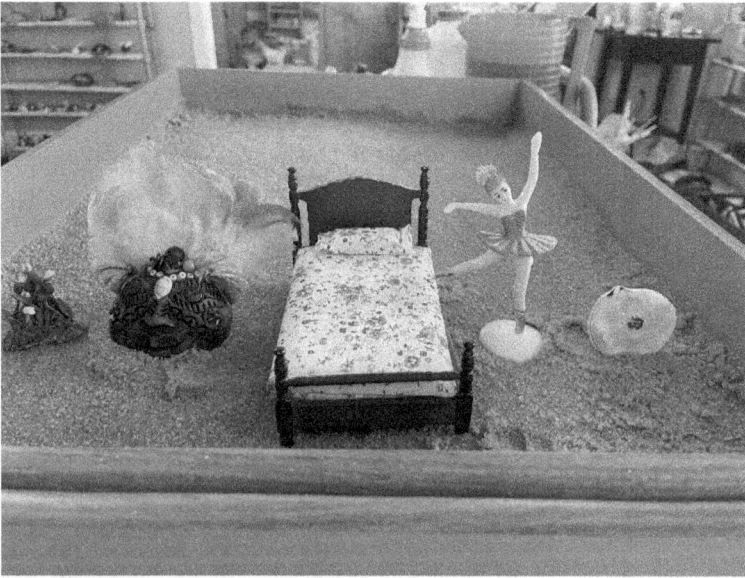

Figure 14.10 Zen Figures Displayed in a Row in the First Tray

Photo by the author

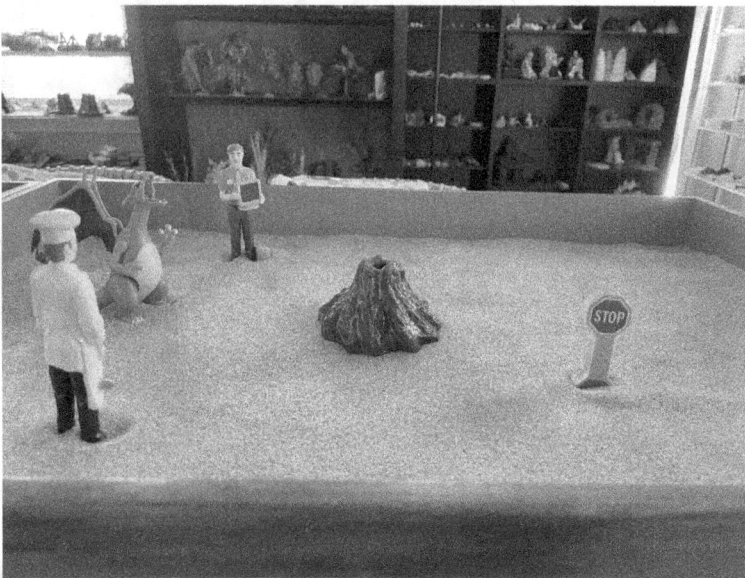

Figure 14.11 Client View of Problem Tray

Photo by the author

9. Check in with the client and ask them how and where they feel sensations in their body. Validate their responses.

10. Ask the client there is more they want to say about the tray or what is happening in their body.

11. If the clinician is going to incorporate the modality of EMDR, inform the client this is going to be the next step in the process.

12. Show the client the portable EMDR equipment, a hand-held device and the pulsers which are often referred to as "tactiles."

    a. Inform the client that EMDR utilizes both hemispheres of the brain, and when used in the IFS/Zen/EMDR IFSsandtray both hemispheres are working in conjunction with each other. EMDR appears to assist the client's processing in a gentle way.

    b. Inform the client about the various speeds available when used for processing. The faster speeds will be used at first and the slower speeds are utilized when the client is feeling better about the problem.

13. An example of an EMDR hand-held machine and the pulsers are shown in Figure 14.12.

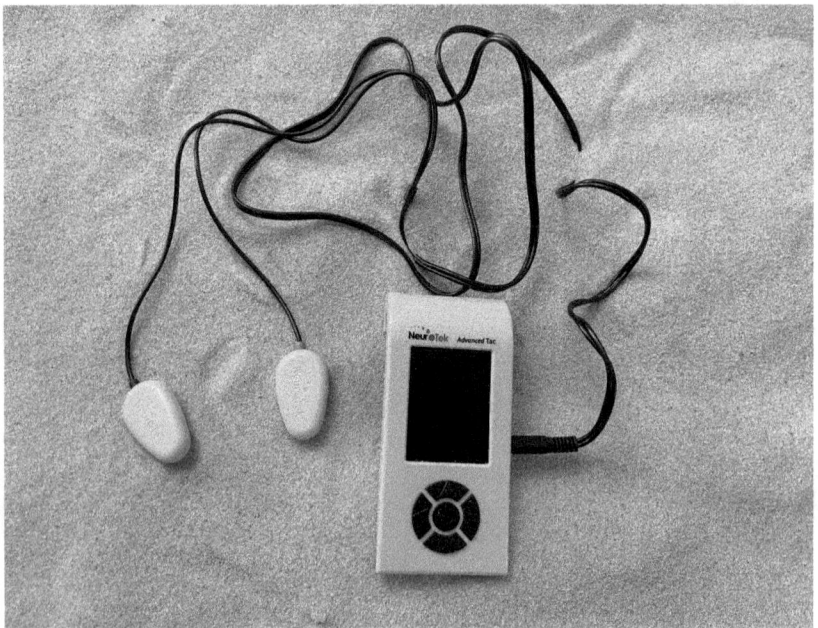

Figure 14.12 Tactile (Pulsers) and EMDR Hand-Held Device

Photo by the author

14. Clinician informs the client they are going to hand them the pulsers under the table, asking to place one tactile under each thigh so the client's hands will be free to move the miniatures they have placed in the trays.
    a. If the client has never used or seen the pulsers, have them hold the tactiles in their hands and tell them you will turn the pulsers on so they can feel what the sensations will feel like when placed under their thighs.
    b. Explain to the client the pulsers are going to be turned on when they are ready. Then, ask for permission, and turn on the pulsers.
15. Once this is completed, ask the client to put the pulsers under their thighs, but don't turn pulsers on yet.
16. Ask the client if they could rate, on a scale of zero to ten, how upsetting it is for them to see the problem tray. Ranking it at a zero if it is not a problem and up to a ten if the issue is very upsetting.
    a. Ask them if they currently notice any body sensations as well.
17. Inform the client you are going to turn the pulsers on and find a speed that works for the client.
    a. Once the speed is approved by the client, begin processing.
18. Have the client spend one to two minutes looking at the problem tray. Check-in with them, and if they respond it isn't too upsetting, ask them to look at it a little longer.
19. When the client says to the clinician it is upsetting, ask them to look at the Zen figures and remind you what these figures represented to the client.
    a. This will bring the client back to a calmer state.
20. Inform the client they can have both Zen feelings and hold the problem at the same time. (Ask the client to move the Zen figures and place them into the problem tray where the Zen figure is most needed.) See Figure 14.13.
21. Ask the client what they are noticing as they place the Zen figures into the problem tray.
22. After a few moments, inform the client their hands are free to move the tray in any way if they want to change it.
    a. Use the words, "I am wondering if anything in this tray now needs to be moved around or taken out of the tray."
23. Inform the client if anything wants to be taken out of the tray and won't be used again, place it into the container. If they feel they may need the miniature again, to just place it in the other tray. Note: in the photograph of Betty's tray the volcano was placed out to the scene and in the other tray (see Figure 14.14).

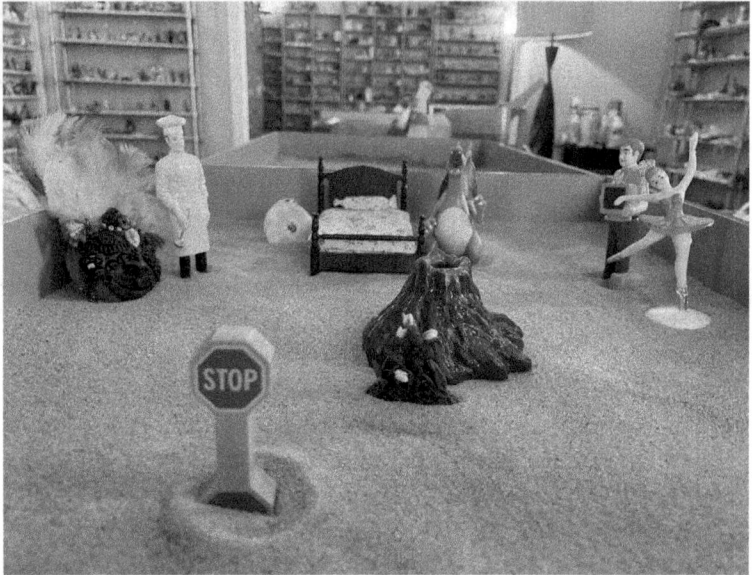

Figure 14.13 Client View of Zen Figures Placed into the Problem Tray

Photo by the author

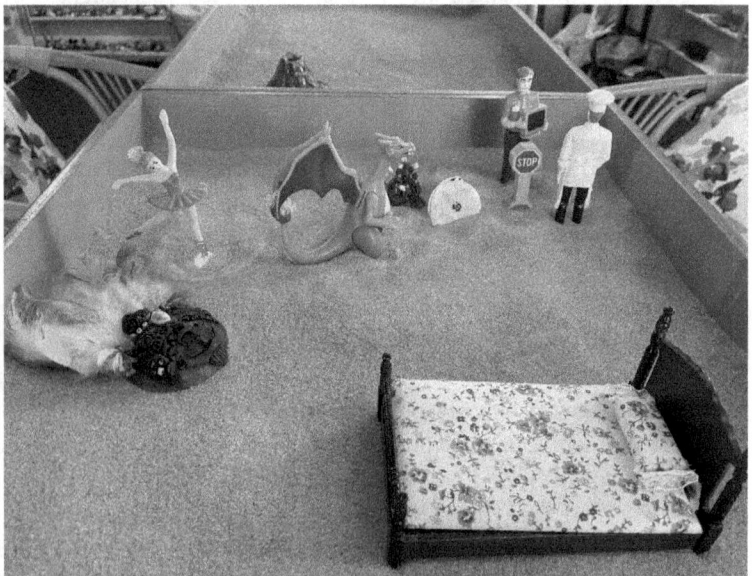

Figure 14.14 Problem Tray with Zen Figures Added

Photo by the author

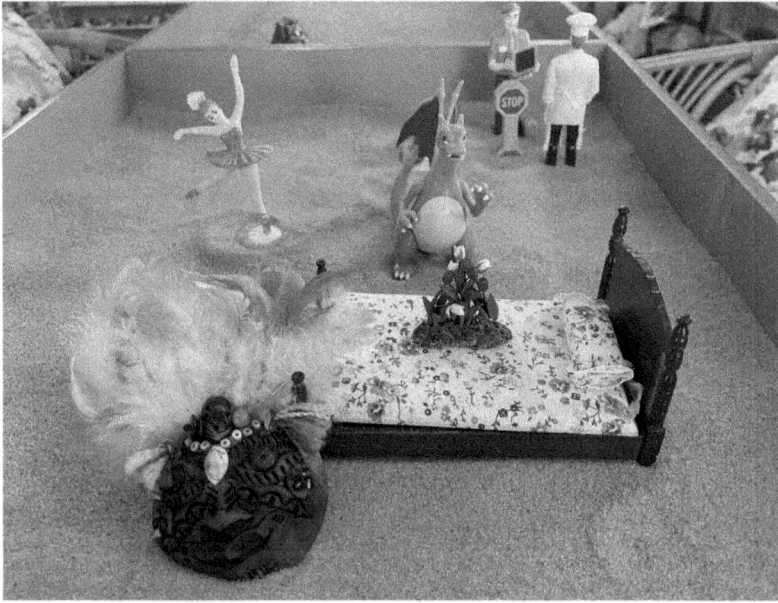

Figure 14.15 Zen Figures Added to Problem Tray

Photo by the author

24. Let the client talk about the new problem tray and how it changed. Continue processing by asking the client to continue viewing the problem tray.
25. Ask the client if the tray needs to change again.
26. Check if any of the miniatures need more Zen assistance. Encourage them to move any of the Zen figures where they are needed (see Figure 14.15).
27. Notice in Betty's tray above how she placed Zen figures near the problematic miniatures.
    a. Betty identified herself as the dragon, a protector of her grandchildren, and how angry it was.
28. If the client identifies with a specific miniature, the clinician should now change to their language directing towards the miniature, "What does the dragon or protector need from the Zen figures to have it feel calmer?"
    a. At this point Betty said, "The dragon needs to go out to the garden, putter around, and forget the world is there." She then moved the flowers to the dragon's side.
29. When the client identifies with the miniature, as Betty did with the dragon, ask the client to close their eyes. Then ask if it feels safe, imagine what it would be like to be the dragon in the garden.

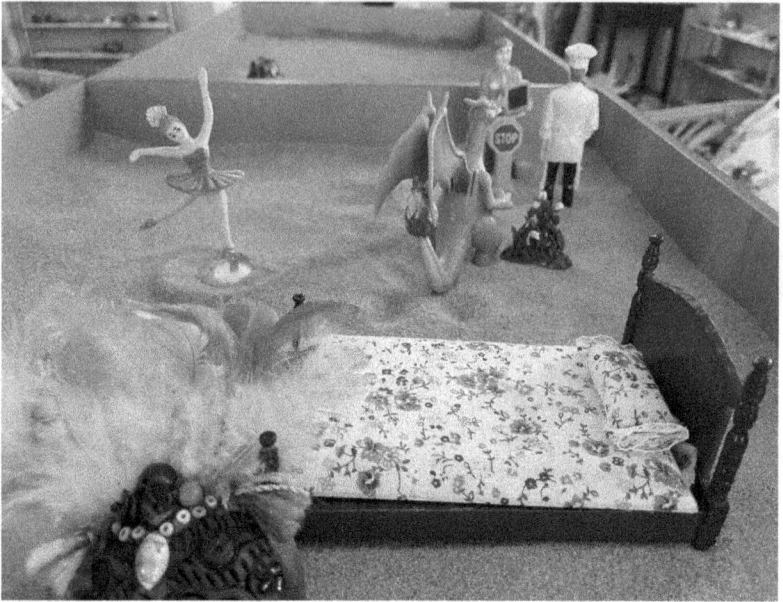

Figure 14.16 Angry Part (Dragon) Receiving Help from the Zen Figure of Flowers

Photo by the author

   a.   The clinician should be creative and repeat back to the client how the Zen figures made them feel. See Figure 14.16.
30. Check in with the client and ask what they are noticing happening in their body.
   a.   Many clients will report calmness at this time.
31. Ask the client how the tray might need to change. See Figure 14.17.
32. Clinician wonders how the angry Part (dragon in the above tray) might handle the situation now that it is in a calm state. See what will help the Part observe and approach the situation differently in a calm way.
   a.   Let the client know they can go back to the stored miniatures and select what Part may help it to remain in a calm state. (Betty chose fire to help her remain calm.)
   b.   Stop EMDR and see Figure 14.18.
33. Ask the client what happens when the Part uses the added miniature. In the picture above the dragon needed to blow off steam with fire.
34. Ask the client what the Part needs after it "blows off steam."
35. The client will know but, if they don't know, say, "I wonder, if you did know what it would be or the Part of you that does know, find that miniature."

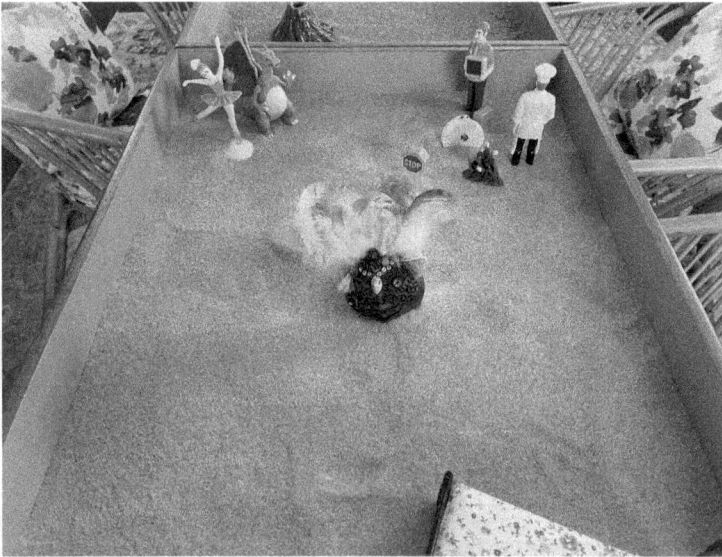

Figure 14.17 Angry Part Joins Zen Figures and Bed Moves Further Back in The Tray

Photo by the author

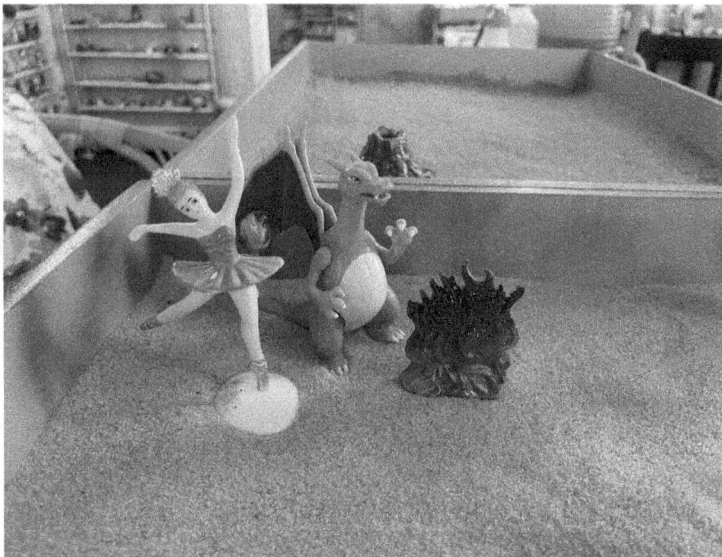

Figure 14.18 A Calm Dragon Blows Off Steam and a Fire Miniature Added

Photo by the author

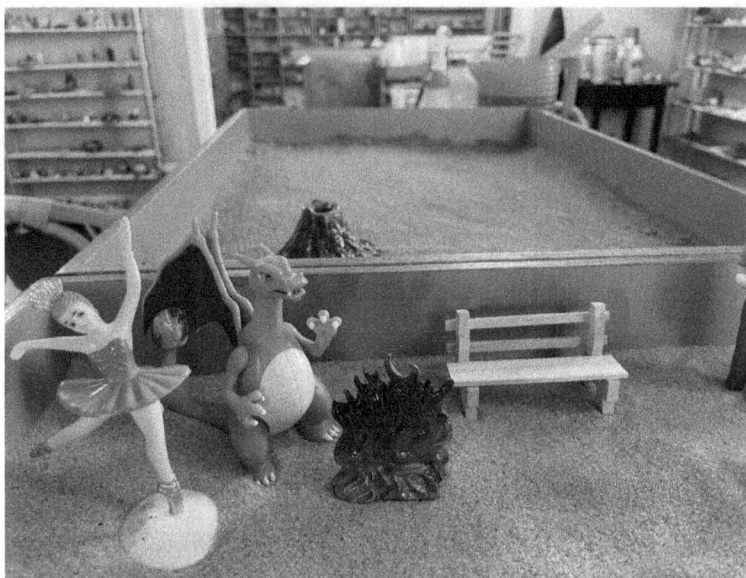

Figure 14.19 Bench Added for the Part to Take a Few Resting Moments

Photo by the author

36. The statement above allows the Part of the client that does know to step in (see Figure 14.19).
37. Check time.
38. Give the client notice when the session is coming to a close and you want to check in with how they are feeling in their body and how does it feel since they first started.
39. Check in with clients to evaluate if they are calm or still upset. Ask them on the zero to ten scale how upset they are now.
    a. If the number is zero have the client check the sensations which coincide with the zero.
    b. If the number is not zero, but lower ask the client to pick up and hold the Zen figures in their hands, if it feels safe, close their eyes, and take a few moments to feel the Zen figures in their hands.
    c. Ask the client to imagine just being in the Zen state and when they are ready open their eyes.
40. Ask the client does the tray need to change in any way.
41. Ask the client to take any miniatures that are no longer needed out of tray and place in the container. See Figure 14.20.
42. Ask client to make the tray in the way as they want it to be now. See Figure 14.21.

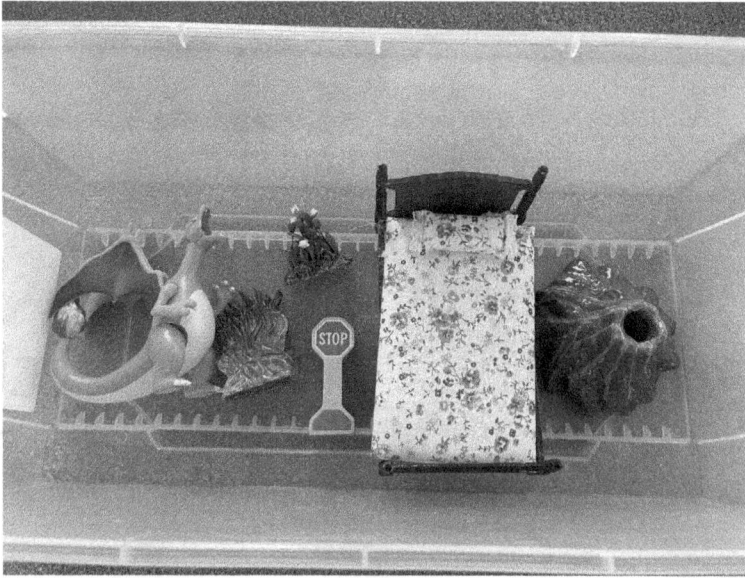

Figure 14.20 Miniatures Removed from the Tray

Photo by the author

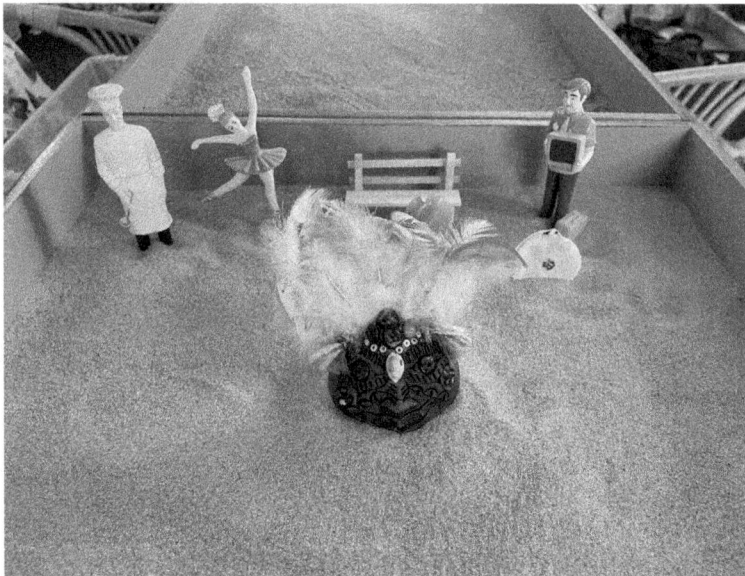

Figure 14.21 Final Tray

Photo by the author

Once completed check in with the client and ask them how they may be able to handle the situation differently now or how they view the problem currently.

In both directives listed above the clinician may find they would like to change a detail or two, due to the knowledge of their client's way of working. The clinician can adjust the session accordingly. This may alter how the exercise proceeds, but when the clinician remains curious and confident, they are in Self in the IFS model/ventral vagal in the PVT. and they may notice this creativity and trust themselves with these new variations.

How to Use the   **15**
Pro-Symptom
Belief Cards with or
without Miniatures

In Chapter 9, "Betty: Healing Early Childhood Trauma with the Pro-Symptom Belief Cards" you were introduced to Betty, who found a new way to address her feelings of inadequacy in just under 40 minutes by using the Pro-Symptom Belief Cards. [I designed the cards which are based on the work of Dr. Francine Shapiro, Dr. Richard Schwartz, Dr. Pat Ogden, Dr. Milton Erikson, Dr. Bruce Ecker, neuroscientists, the non-pathological theories of Dr. Stephen Porges' Polyvagal Theory, and Dr. Bruce Perry's Neurosequential Model of Therapeutics.]

This chapter introduces the reader to incorporating and utilizing the PSBC in their sessions, a brief history of how the cards were developed, and how they relate to what neuroscientists describe as the Default Mode Network (DMN). DMN thoughts can be destructive, and clients may carry adverse core beliefs about themselves which bring them to therapy.

History of the Pro-Symptom Belief Cards

Any reader who has been trained in Eye Movement Desensitization Reprocessing (EMDR) may be familiar with many of the statements found on these cards. Some of the statements are what Dr. Francine Shapiro, founder of EMDR, referred to as "negative cognitions." In Coherence therapy, the work of Dr. Bruce Ecker and his colleagues, these beliefs are called pro-symptom schemas. Somatic work, which focuses on bodily sensations, is a fundamental aspect of working with the PSBC. This type of psychological

DOI: 10.4324/9781003388302-18

work is based on the somatic modalities of Dr. Pat Ogden the founder of Sensorimotor Psychotherapy.

In Greek mythology the Gods and Goddesses Artemis and Apollo are protectors of the young as in the IFS modality protective Parts called Managers and Firefighters. This becomes important for those clinicians who work with metaphor or in the sand with figurines. I realized these cards were recognized as IFS's protectors, Managers, and Firefighters, which are often very young Parts, as described in Dr. Richard Schwartz's Internal Family Systems (IFS) model. These Parts formed when the individual was a child. That person may have experienced upsetting events, early childhood trauma, mis-attunement from their adult caretaker(s) or other major stressors.

The work of Dr. Bruce Perry brings to light how mis-attunement and other factors may result in the development of Parts, as detailed in the IFS model. In the 2009 issue of the *Journal of Loss and Trauma*, Perry writes,

> … the malleability of the brain shifts during development, and there for the timing and specific "pattern" of neglect influence the final functional outcome. A child deprived of consistent, attentive, and attuned nurturing for the first 3 years of life who is then adopted and begins to receive attention, love, and nurturing may not be capable of benefiting from these experiences with the same malleability as an infant. In some cases, this later love is insufficient to overcome the dysfunctional organization of the neural systems mediating socioemotional interactions.

In Perry's statement above, he notes if a child is deprived of a consistent, attentive, and attuned nurturing adult in the first three years of life, the child can and will often experience dysfunctional organization of the neural systems in the brain later in life. In IFS this correlates with how often the protective Parts will identify themselves as the age of ten and younger. These Parts are known as Exiles in IFS. Exiles are the Parts frozen in time at the age the individual experienced the upsetting or traumatic event. Frequently, Exiles can be even younger than the age of four.

When a person experiences difficulty in early childhood, that individual's DMN will link the past with the present in adulthood where core perceptions are negative. Dr. Jeffrey Rediger, in his 2020 book, *Cured: The Life-Changing Science of Spontaneous Healing*, writes,

> We interpret the things that happen to us in our unique way and "record" events the way we perceive them. When we go back over these events in our minds, as we all tend to do with significant things (especially if

they're negative or we experienced them intensely), we activate the DMN repeatedly in the same patterns, creating neural pathways with deepening "grooves" over time ... Neuroscientist have nicknamed it the *me network*. It's the neurobiological basis of the self; *it's who you are.*

(p. 270)

Basically, the DMN is located in the midbrain, mainly in the medial prefrontal cortex, and the posterior cingulate cortex. The prefrontal cortex is in the middle of the brain nearer the forehead, whereas the posterior cingulate cortex is positioned closer to the back of the brain, also in the middle range. The DMN is a reflective process, happens when a person isn't involved in a task, and the mind of the client appears to be wandering. When the DMN is activated along with other regions of the brain, human beings are likely to wonder about themselves (Seigel 2018).

Working with Pro-Symptom Belief Cards

Prior to the first session, the clinician asks a client to fill out a brief questionnaire which includes listing six qualities, three strengths, and three limitations. In the first meeting, the clinician maintains curiosity about what the client described as their presenting difficulties and these six beliefs, especially the limitations. It is important to pay close attention to what each individual perceives as their shortcomings. Often in that first appointment or the next, the clinician asks the client if they might like to try an experiential exercise to learn a little bit more about the limiting beliefs they carry. The clients are often very curious and customarily agree to explore these often-undesirable, self-identified imperfections, and gain an understanding of where they stem.

In the first or second session, ask the client to focus on the concerns, distress, or trepidations which brought them into therapy. The clinician begins by asking the client if they are interested in finding out a little bit more about the presenting issue and might like to try an experiential exercise. If the client agrees, follow the guidelines, which are listed in sequential order.

1. Inform the client this experiential exercise may take approximately 10 to 15 minutes and will be an exploration into where they may have learned the beliefs.
2. Explain to the client you are going to ask them to think about the presenting issue, look at the PSBC, and pick cards that feel true about themselves when they are experiencing the presenting issue

3. The clinician may begin with, *"I am going to get up and give you a set of laminated cards. They are call Pro-Symptom Belief Cards, there are twenty-five in the deck, and each one has a statement which may not seem positive, such as 'I am not good enough', 'I am inadequate,' and other core beliefs which many human beings have in adulthood. If there is another belief that you have, please let me know what that maybe. What we are going to do is have you focus your body when you think about the presenting problem and the beliefs that you feel about yourself at that time."*

   a. Inform the client by saying, (After you say the words above and allowing the client to prepare for the clinician to enter their space, allowing the body to be less reactive.) "I want to let you know your autonomic nervous systems (ANS) is just getting used to this space, me, and any movements I make might be perceived as threatening to the ANS. The ANS is part of your own body's defense system, and I'll explain more about that next session. Will that be okay with that?"

   b. If the client wants more information about their ANS, the clinician should agree and say, "Okay, today I will spend the session telling you more about the ANS. We will do the experiential exercise next time."

   c. If they don't need to know, continue the exercise.

4. What the clinician is about to learn is whether the client can connect with their body sensations or not. It is also an introduction for the client to understand how sensations are connected to core beliefs, which brought them into therapy.

   a. If the client can connect with their body the exercise is likely to be successful.

   b. If they can't connect with their body, the individual is a candidate for another modality. The clinician will decide which therapeutic tool they want to use, such as working with the unconscious with Kalffian sandplay or IFSsandtray, art therapy, Trauma-Informed Cognitive Behavioral Therapy, etc. … Using a modality that can access the unconscious is best. [Add something like: there is no right or wrong here. Be sure to assure your client that you have other exercises that might feel better for them at this time.]

5. Say to the client, "This exercise may or may not work today as we have just met, but it will be very informative in how I will work with you going forward. It will also assist me in determining what the best modality I know to assist you in your healing. Are you willing to give it a try?"

   a. Generally, the client will be very interested and want to learn more about themselves and will say yes.

6. Clinician you can say to the client, I am going to get up now and hand you the cards. What I want you to do is close your eyes if it feels safe enough to do so or focus on a point on the wall behind me during the experience. I will let you know when to close your eyes. The reason I will ask you to close your eyes is because there are a lot of visually stimulating things in this office that you may find distracting. Closing your eyes will allow you to concentrate on any sensations happening within your body, but before we do the experiential, I am going to ask you to think about the presenting issues that brought you in today.

7. Get up and give them the set of cards and return to your seat.

8. Tell the client, "Are you ready to begin? Go through all of the cards, put the ones you feel true about yourself in one pile and the ones that don't feel true in another pile."

   a. The clinician waits and watches the client closely without saying a word, unless the client asks the clinician a question.

9. Once the client has finished, the clinician can ask the client to place the cards which didn't fit on the table or the surface next to them.

10. Have the client put the ones that fit on the floor in front of them by color in a vertical row so they can see all the statements. There are four colors: black, blue, lime green, and white.

11. Ask the client to tell you what beliefs they pick by looking at the cards at their feet. Starting with the row on the left and moving to the right.

12. Have the client narrow it down to one row of colored cards, either black, blue, lime green or white.

    a. The black cards represent beliefs that are protective Parts carrying burdens of control and choice.

    b. The blue are beliefs protective Parts carrying burdens of safety or vulnerability.

    c. The lime green are beliefs protective Parts carrying burdens of responsibility.

    d. The white are protective Parts carrying burdens of self-defectiveness.

13. Have the client narrow it down to one card from the remaining row. Based on the color, this will also narrow the scope of the Protective Part involved.

14. Ask the client to get as comfortable as possible and inform them you will be taking notes.

15. Ask the client what the belief is and write it down and tell the client they can now place the card next to the other cards they didn't pick.

16. Inform the client you would like them to close their eyes or look at a point on the wall behind you.

17. Once the client has closed their eyes or is focused on a point in the wall, ask them to focus on the card and the issue that brought them into therapy or the triggering event.

18. Ask the client to notice the internal sensations in their body and give a menu listed below:

    a. The menu of sensations can be a knot in your stomach, something in tightness in your throat, a weight on your chest, or something in your stomach like a pit, and it can also be a tingling sensation, tell them to just notice the slightest sensation.

19. When the client responds with a sensation, ask them to describe what that sensation feels like in their body.

    a. If the client has difficulty after giving the menu this may be an individual who has disconnected from the body and there may be another modality the clinician will have to utilize instead of the cards.

    b. Try for just a few more minutes to continue the exercise, but if the client is unable to connect with their body sensations, have them open their eyes and reassure them they did a great job. At this point, you know another modality will be used.

20. When the client informs the clinician, they feel a sensation of _____, it could be a heaviness in their chest, for example, ask them what that heaviness feels like as a weight.

    a. The clinician asks the client if it is like a one-pound, two-pound, or heavier weight, or a sensation of pressure on the chest.

    b. Or if the sensation is of tightness in their throat, ask them if it's like an elastic ball, squeezing sensation, etc. ... The idea is to get a complete understanding of what they're describing.

21. Ask the client to focus on the scene of being triggered, and the sensation they described, while they think about the presenting problem. Throughout, they are keeping their eyes closed.

    a. Inform the client they can do both: focus on the sensation and the scene or triggering event.

    b. Ask when they felt the same identical sensations before their current age, (name their age). Repeat one or two times, adding, "Just focus on those sensations as if that's the only thing you have to focus on right now. Is there a scene or image that pops up and don't edit whatever comes up is the right thing, just let me know. Just focus on the same heaviness you are feeling now and when did you feel the same identical sensations before the age of _____?" The blank is the client's current age.

22. The client will come up with a younger age and scene.

23. Ask the client to focus on that younger age, the sensations of _____ (heaviness), and the new scene at the younger age. Repeat number 19 above until they come to another younger age.
    a.   If they can't come to another age tell them to open their eyes and reassure them like in step 19.
    b.   If they do have a scene or memory say, "That's right."
24. Ask the client what new scene or memory that has just popped up. Ask them to see themselves in that scene now, as if now is then and then is now. (This is called the confusion technique in hypnosis) and repeat "Focus on your body sensations again as if now is then and then is now." Have them focus on the same heaviness or another emotion at the same time. Give the client time and reassure them with comforting words. If the clinician has to repeat step 19, do so. The client will come up with a younger age and scene.
25. Say to the client, "You can focus on that younger scene as if you are in that younger scene now. What is happening with the heaviness and just notice any other sensations in another part of your body with this new scene?" The clinician should repeat number 19.
26. The clinician asks what scene or memory popped up? It will be younger than the last scene or memory.
27. The client will often have another scene pop up that is another younger age. Repeat number 19 or 20? and if the client can't come up with another scene, then ask the client to open their eyes.
28. Congratulate the client for a successful ability to trust their body sensations.
29. Explain to the client what they just did informs you. This technique should be a successful way to help them heal from the aspects of themselves, or Parts, that carry burdens from when they were younger.
30. Explain to the client this technique is one way you can work.
31. Let them know the starting pro-symptom belief is tied into the younger memories or scenes that popped up and the trigger most likely will be younger than the last scene.
32. Inform the client due to the few minutes allocated to use in this session it was just a quick experiential exercise to understand if this would be a technique for you to use to heal them.

When a client can do this experiential exercise, they are usually very excited to get their therapy work started. They will find utilizing body sensations easy and will most likely find working with their Parts much easier. As discussed in this book, Parts have bodies too, are frozen in time, and, when accessed somatically. exiled Parts will show up. This allows the clinician to heal the Parts which will let go of burdens resulting in healing the exiled Part, the protective Parts, and the client will carry a newfound positive belief.

Working with Pro-Symptom Belief Cards with Miniatures

If you are a clinician who has a sandtray and miniatures, you will be able to externalize the Part of the person that has a pro-symptom belief. Make sure you have discussed the IFS model and the role of protectors and have had the client do the introduction to IFS/PVT IFSsandtray experiential from Chapter 14.

1. Give the cards to the client and ask them to think about an upsetting or triggering event. Ask the client to pick as many of the cards that feel true about themselves when they think about the triggering situation or event.
2. Ask the client to arrange the cards by color and narrow it down to one set.
3. Ask the client to find the one card in that set that feels the truest about themselves and connects with a sensation in their body.
4. Have the client find a miniature that best represents the card they just picked.
5. Have them put it in the center of the tray facing toward themselves.
6. Tell the client this is the Part of themselves that feels (whatever belief the client has picked.)
7. Say to the client, *"This is a Part of you that feels _____. (Fill in the blank with the belief) I think it has messages for you. This Part of you is now represented by the miniature you picked that is in the center of the tray and now is externalized. This is the Part of you that feels."*
8. It is going to be a pro or reactive Part known as the Protectors (Managers or Firefighters) in IFS.
9. Say to the client, *"This is a one of the Protectors that is responding to the situation you picked from the cards. It was triggering to you or made you upset. This Part is showing up when the situation and pro-symptom belief are held together. We're going to find out more information about how this Part is trying to help you because all emotions and all Parts have positive intents."*
10. Point to the miniature in the tray and say, *"This miniature represents the Part of you that has a positive intent, or reason, and it's trying to help you.*

It's one of the Protectors we discussed earlier when we discussed the proactive and reactive Parts in IFS. Now, just as a refresher, can you tell me what the Protectors do?"

11. Let the client tell you what they know about their proactive and reactive Parts that you addressed in the IFS/PVT IFSsandtray. Gently remind them of what they did in the that sandtray if they need assistance.

12. Ask the client to find a figure to represent Self, or their calm state.

13. Have the client place the Self figure into the tray.

14. Have the client tell you what about the Self figure makes them feel in their body and how it helps keep them in calm or in the ventral vagal state.

15. Ask the client to notice how calm they feel in their body when they see the miniature that they picked for Self, externalized in the sand tray before them.

    a. When the client feels calm, it is highly likely they are in the ventral vagal state which is Self in IFS (calm, clarity, courage, compassionate, connected, confident, and shows curiosity).

    b. If the client needs to hold the miniature, ask them to pick it up and hold it, and ask what they notice happening in their body as sensations.

16. Tell the client they can hold both the Self calm feelings as well as the triggered feelings at the same time. Tell the client you are about to ask them to talk and act as if they were both miniatures. Tell them they can be calm when they talk for the figure representing Self and respond as though they are triggered when they are acting like the other figure, which is most likely a reactive Part or Firefighter in IFS.

    • If the client has difficulties at the point most likely a skeptical or concerned Part that has questions that have not been addressed. If this occurs the clinician should check in with Part by asking it what it's concerned about.

17. Ask the client what the Self figure would say to the triggered protective Part in the tray to help it.

18. Then have the client respond as if they are the triggered Part.

    a. This is like doing the Gestalt empty chair technique: the clinician asks the client to imagine a person they are having difficulty with sitting in an empty chair and engage in an emotional dialog with the other individual.

    b. In this case the client is having a dialog with their Part from Self.

19. End the session when the client can do this for a few moments

20. Congratulate the client for a successful ability to be in both roles.

Once this experiential is completed, the clinician can be creative and work with triggered Parts in the tray and bring in the client's Self as an externalized Part.

Resources

Perry, B., "Examining childhood maltreatment through a neurodevelopmental lens: Clinical applications of the neurosequential model of therapeutics," *Journal of Loss and Trauma*, 2009. https://doi.org/10.1080/15325020903004350

Rediger, J., *Cured: The life-changing science of spontaneous healing*. Flatiron Books, New York, NY, 2020 (p. 270).

Siegel, D., *Aware: The science and practice of presence the groundbreaking meditation practice*. Mind Your Brain, Inc. Random House LLC, New York, NY, 2018 (pp. 135–137).

Section Four

Outcomes of Client's Healing Expeditions

Soul Reflections   **16**
Discovery of Self-Acceptance

I don't believe it's me who heals my clients. I believe they are the instrument for all healing. I even tell them the body was designed to heal itself. For example, recently I was doing the dishes and I didn't see the newly sharpened knife in the water. Unknowingly, I reached through the suds and sliced my finger. There was a considerable amount of blood and thought I might need stitches. I bandaged my finger and staunched the bleeding. The next morning, when I was changing the dressing, I saw that it was already healing. The body knows how to heal itself. We just have to be present, apply the right bandages, so to speak, and allow it to do its job. The body knows how to do that. The psyche has the capacity to heal the mind—in much the same way—by using the unconscious.

When some of my clients found out I was writing a book, they couldn't wait to share *what happened to them*. They understood the power of their unconscious to heal themselves. They all learned their behavior was a result of early childhood trauma, upsetting events, or growing up in a chaotic environment. All of them said the same thing, "If you can help just one person who suffered like me, I want you to use my story, the images of my trays, and words." They felt and knew how important their healing was and wanted to help others in the way they felt I helped them.

I told them all in the very first session, "it's going to be you who will heal yourself, not me." These clients are really my co-therapists. I give them credit when they trust their unconscious in an unknown process. It was a huge leap of faith for all of them. It was all about trust. Leona said in Chapter 17, "trust is hard once you have trauma."

DOI: 10.4324/9781003388302-20

In the cases of John and Billy who were deemed "sex addicts," they sought comfort in out of control sexual behavior. The "sex addiction" label doesn't help anyone suffering from a dysregulated and sympathetically aroused system. In the case of Billy, even his couple's therapist pigeon-holed him. He was a sex addict and that's all there was to it: he was damaged. I knew we could address the behavior by learning about the trauma, and understanding how he had come to use sex to escape or to soothe his wounded parts. Sadly, people who carry labels—stark pronouncements from a professional—come to believe they are indeed, what they have been diagnosed with, further diminishing their capacity to heal. The labels mask the truth, the underlying childhood trauma, further propelling the individuals into the fight or flight state. This is dangerous.

In all the cases I have shared, misdiagnoses from professionals who may not know about the Polyvagal Theory, not even asking how the individual survived in their family of origin. When I think of John from Chapter 4, who received a diagnosis of ADHD, it makes me wonder about all of the children in the world who have been labeled with whatever prevailing diagnosis was popular at the time. Did the professional who diagnosed them ask about early childhood trauma? Or the history of trauma that may have been generational? I will never know the answer to that question.

Jane—featured in Chapters 12 and 13—said that meeting her parts in IFSsandtray changed her life. She recently checked in with me, astounded that she could now achieve multiple orgasms. Having suffered from vaginismus, she couldn't believe how far she had come. She shared an intimate conversation she had with her partner David before working in the sand. I asked her to write it down so I could share it in the book.

Jane wanted to share her story of how she and David had two major conversations. One, when they realized they wanted to share a life together, and the other, after her therapy with me was finished. She expresses it better than I ever could.

> Before IFSsandtray therapy with you: The situation I was in was heartbreaking, frustrating, and bittersweet. I am so in love with my partner David but felt like I was being unfair to him. I was certain that I will never be able to have intercourse with him. When David and I began our relationship, we talked about the fact that we could do other things, but actual penetration was off the table. Even my gynecologist said it was highly unlikely. I remember the night we were sitting by the fire, and with tears in my eyes.
>
> I said to him, "Would you be able to just hold my hand, if it came to that, like…forever?" He said, "Absolutely, we are worth it. I love you."

This was incredibly meaningful to me. I wish from the bottom of my heart that I could be with him in this most intimate of ways. I feel just horrible.

Here is the second aspect of that email:

After IFSsandtray therapy with you: This morning David and I were holding hands after having intercourse in the most amazing, intimate, and meaningful way. He looked at me and said, "Would you be able to just hold my hand, if it came to that, like...forever?" I looked at him quizzically, and said, "Of course, but what are you talking about?"

"That's what you said to me nine months ago. And I absolutely would have been fine with that. Just look how far we've come. I love you so much."

"Then,", with a sly smile, he said "And THIS is so much better!"

She added at the very end the following, which I thought was so sweet and speaks to her humbleness.

For the last line, I don't know if it should be included, or if I should say "incredible" instead of "better." I don't want it to seem as if sex is the be all/end all.

I hope you agree, she said it better.

I love being a therapist, and I would never ask anyone to do what I haven't done. I have been in your shoes, whether you are a therapist in the role of a healer, or as a client who wants alignment. I only ask that you come with me and trust the process. I will hold your hand. Let me be the rope to keep you safe. Together, we will take this journey.

Client's Reflections of Their Self-Acceptance with In-Depth Therapy

17

Of course, when my clients showed interest in being included in my book, my first thoughts were about client confidentiality. I can't truly summarize the extent of my practice in these few examples of case studies. However, while researching this work, I reached out to several other clients to get their overall assessment of the process and our work together. I've excepted some of these stories below to show you a cross-section of the types of issues I've encountered, and the various success stories that were a result of working with the unconscious.

Reflections from a Satisfied Couple

Grace and William (pseudonyms) originally come to me in hopes of gaining clarity when they navigated their swinging lifestyle. Like all human beings, individuals who are in the lifestyle, have Parts. If a person isn't aware of their own vulnerable Parts that individual's protective Parts will engage. This could be a Manager, but often it is a Firefighter. This reactive Part is most likely going to defend the person from experiencing the wounded Exile Part. Often when the reactive Firefighter takes over the individual will become angry or defensive and not be able to engage with their significant other.

Like many therapists who see couples, I'd seen them both together and individually for a few sessions throughout the therapy when needed. I knew their experiences were key to help illustrate these therapeutic approaches.

DOI: 10.4324/9781003388302-21

William had worked in the sand first in a few of his individual sessions. I learned Grace would always ask him when he got home, "How was your session? What are you learning about yourself, us, and what happened when you worked in the sand? Describe it to me?"

He couldn't, admitting to me, "I can't explain any of this to Grace because I can't put it into words; because of that Grace doesn't think I am really trying to heal. She also feels that I don't know how much I have hurt her by what I had done when I betrayed her. I do know. I love her; I am changing and will never hurt her like that again."

His enthusiasm about his experiences working in the sand was infectious, so I asked Grace if she wouldn't mind writing something about her own experience. She got back to me later that night. Her level of detail and intricate descriptions of the process and her reaction merit inclusion here:

> I went to see Peg Hurley Dawson with my fiancé for relationship therapy a few years ago and cannot say enough of how much it significantly helped us with our relationship, even more as individuals. William and I have been through a lot over the past ten years including cheating, lying, and unexpectedly losing our beautiful dog Teddy. I never thought the weight I was carrying could ever be lifted.

> I had been to a few therapists in the past where I sat down on a couch for an hour and told the therapist all my problems. At the time I thought I felt better after a session since I verbally talked about my feelings to someone. I never experienced any physical change throughout my body. After my first few visits with Peg, she introduced us to sandplay, showed us this room filled with an overwhelming number of random figurines and trinkets.

> It was very intimidating to say the least! At my next session alone, Peg asked if I wanted to give it a try. She explained how I would go around the room and pick different items up and place them in whatever way I wanted to in this sandbox in the middle of the room. Skeptical is an understatement of how I felt at this point. I didn't know who was crazier, my therapist or me. I decided to put my skepticism aside and give this "sandbox" thing a shot. I walked around the room, I remember wanting to laugh at myself and even roll my eyes at what I was doing, thinking this is the dumbest thing I have ever done at thirty-three years old, playing with toys in a sandbox.

> Although it was extremely hard, I tried to be as optimistic as possible. I walked around the room trying to think of how I would arrange these

items that I had chosen. I still did not understand how this could possibly help me and my relationship with William. I assembled my pieces in the sandbox and kept staring at it, and after looking at what I made, I got quite emotional. I was extremely touched by what I had created, and I was just looking at this silly sandbox artwork I had made.

The best way I can describe how I felt after leaving that first session was as though I walked in wearing a backpack full of books that I have been lifelessly carrying around with me for such a long time. Almost instantaneous when I walked out of her office, I felt as though someone secretly took out several of those books to make what I was carrying so much lighter. The feeling I felt throughout my body was so significant I cried. I didn't even know why I was crying. I didn't even know what had just happened. It was the craziest, most amazing feeling I had felt in a very long time. I felt I had an epiphany.

Although I had all these amazing body sensations and feelings after my first session, I was still a little weary of the whole thing. It still seemed a little wacky that I played in a sandbox for an hour even though it felt so amazing after. How could that be? I knew I had to try it again! I had several more sandplay sessions after that, and I began putting more of my skepticism aside and allowing my mind to relax completely.

I think it is important to note, Grace's skepticism was a Part. That Part's concerns were valid and by Grace's willingness to go forward the skeptical Part began to trust the sandplay process.

Every single session I had after that was an even more revitalizing experience for me. One of my last sessions was especially memorable for me because I went in dealing with so many relationship issues with my fiancé that I wanted to figure out. I would have thought my sandbox would have reflected that to me. It was amazing how different it was, and so impactful to my current situation. It was the first time I had used both sand trays and both of my masterpieces were incredibly different when viewed side by side, I understood what they meant. It was extremely emotional for me. I came to realize that everything I was feeling on the outside was really triggered by something so much deeper on the inside that I never was consciously aware of, or feelings that had been so far suppressed I assumed they were gone, and I was over them. You would think that after an experience like this it would just bring back bad memories and I would become sad or angry, it was the complete opposite. I felt more powerful and stronger than before I walked through her door.

I have talked to many close friends about my sandplay therapy and how it has helped me, I always seem to get that skeptical "you're crazy" look because it is so difficult to explain in words just how life changing sandplay therapy truly is. Sandplay therapy goes so incredibly deep— deeper than anything I have ever experienced, and you don't even realize it! It has been by far the most impactful type of therapy I have ever done.

I can honestly say that sandplay therapy significantly changed my life for the better. Not only for my relationship, and as an individual. My life has completely uplifted in ways that I cannot describe in words. I could not believe how fast it can happen too. It has truly saved my life and I will be forever grateful.

More Reflections

Leona had been seeing me for three years. She initially came to me because I am a sex therapist who specializes in working with the kink community, couples, and those with complex trauma. She readily agreed to allow me to record her thoughts for use in my book. I must warn all the readers, she does swear in this explanation. I left it in because she is real; everything she said was real and unvarnished.

When I did the sandtray, it felt weird, once I figured out Parts, those voices in my head, the Parts coming up, and talking. That was like a learning step to trust my inner voice, trust my inner intuition, and trust the things I think about that come to mind, and I could trust myself.

Her use of the word "trust" is significant. As outlined in the introductory chapter, "trust the process" is key to assessing the unconscious. Her reaction to the nonverbal, nondirective sandplay, however, was vastly different.

When we did the first sandplay, I fucking hated it, hated it. This is not for me; I don't know what I am going to do. If this is what Peg's into, maybe we're not a good fit because I don't know what goes on. Not only was it saying you just have to take a leap of faith, and I have to trust that something is happening. Because I couldn't hear it and hold it, it was really difficult to trust it, because I didn't trust it, I didn't believe in it. So, I did the tray and I hated it. I didn't know what it was all about., I don't know if you remember I didn't want to do that anymore. I just went right back to the Parts sandtray.

Then I remembered I signed up for a mystery quilt once. Once a month they would send me black fabric and they said to make fifty squares. The next month they said make eighty orange triangles, etc … So, I was cutting those things and I had no idea what I was making. I cut all the pieces; I had no idea what it was going to be. I didn't know until the very end when they sent me a picture of how to assemble it all. And I said to myself, oh, doing the pieces, doing the process, doing the work all added up to this big, beautiful quilt.

Once I realized that, I remembered you said, "It's not about one tray, but it really happens if you look at the process of the trays." Once I kind of saw that I knew I could have faith in it because I know it's going toward something that I don't see. Just because I don't see it doesn't mean it's not real. Just because I don't know what it's going to look like doesn't mean it's not beautiful. Just because I don't know what size it is, doesn't mean it won't keep me warm.

I don't have to know the fucking answers to that shit. When someone says, "I promise that it's going towards something better. Which in this case instead of a quilt, its mental health, less trauma, less stuck inside the bad stuff. So, I was in control in the sandtray, which I needed because I needed to be in control of something.

You know with trauma it's rare to be in control of anything. In sandplay I had to trust in you as a guide. So, I had to not only trust the process and also when I had to trust in a human being to keep me safe. When you have trauma like me, that's huge.

There's the step of having faith in yourself that what I do—no matter what—is good. That's BIG! That's really BIG! When you have shit on yourself and everything you do, you fuck up and you're a failure, and all of that. And in the tray, no matter what I do even if I put a pile of rocks in the middle of this thing (the tray) and it's perfect. It's okay, it's what should be there. That's HUGE! Just that. Even if the tray did nothing. Just learning that aspect that I am a worthy human and what I do is good or what I do matters no matter what it is. That's cool. Then it's also because I still laugh at myself because I don't know why I pick up the pieces.

At this point I reassured her that nobody knows why they choose the pieces they choose, that is one of the reasons the process works so well. What is happening when working with sandplay is we are accessing the unconscious or the right hemisphere of the brain, which doesn't have language, instead relying on the miniatures as symbols for language.

Because really, when I get in the sandplay room, and I start looking at the pieces, I know I might do it differently than other people because I talk about it more and you don't even have to talk about it. Like you said, "we don't have to figure out what this is." It's just doing it. Sitting with it and accepting that and being able to laugh and cry and feel safe and then leave it. Having the shit you learn in your tray affects your everyday life.

That's why I keep coming back. Something happens. I don't know what it is and it's really hard to describe to people. I say it's kind of like you want to go cave diving. Which is really fucking dangerous, cave diving is dangerous especially when you have been in bad caves. It's your cave, you can go in or not. You pick. The therapist doesn't tell you what the cave is, doesn't tell you what's in the cave, what they're there for is … It's like you said: "I am here if you get stuck, I'm here if you need help, I'm here if you get frozen, and I need to bring you back out, I'm here if you need supplies, and if you went in by yourself, you couldn't explore as far as you can with that kind of backup.

The trust between therapist and client is paramount. Leona's metaphor was apt. I was reminded of my husband's cave diving, and how he depended on a rope to reassure him that he could always find a way out of the cave. My role in this therapy is like that rope: my clients are doing all the hard work, swimming in the deep. I'm there to keep them safe, secure with the knowledge they can always come back. Leona's acceptance of the process and growing passion helped her find a better way of healing. She summarized it best with one of her candid, funny pronouncements.

Later, Leona brought up another aspect of my practice that she found particularly helpful.

How could I overlook your 123-pound therapy dog, Harvey? Harvey just brings everything down to a much more casual level. I love dogs as well. Having him and giving him attention, I find myself saying things that I wouldn't necessarily come forth saying. It's just a relaxing kind of distraction. And he's the best dog. I feel a certain connection when I'm interacting with the dog and for me it's easier to talk. I love it when Harvey is here.

Not all my clients like dogs, and in those cases he's perfectly content to ignore us, splaying himself upside down on the sofa, legs spread, showing his manhood to the world, and taking a break from boring human activities. Throughout my practice, I've seen, again and again, how the simple act of petting Harvey can have a calming, relaxing effect on my clients. In general, animals have a way of bringing an individual into a calm/ventral state.

In order for therapy to really be effective, a client has to feel safe and trust their therapist. It is how we heal, in connection with others which ultimately allows connection with ourselves. This state (ventral vagal) also allows for so many wonderful things to happen such as creativity, confidence, and clarity.

A Message from Cleopatra

Another client, asked me to use the pseudonym from a figure she uses often in her sandplay sessions, Cleopatra.

I had been seeing Cleopatra for a little over two years. She has complex trauma from early childhood experiences, and we use all of the modalities in my therapeutic tool kit. She wrote over three single-spaced pages about her experience of working with me. The following is an excepted from her letter.

What she wrote represented the ventral state:

> Depending on how we started our session with talk therapy or other modalities, or just diving right into working in the sand, each and every time is different and unique. It sounds so weird, like you pick out these characters off a shelf and then play in the sand. Then when you live it and you make a tray and over time you make more and more you realize, you don't pick the characters, they pick you. It's quite beautiful to sit over your completed artwork and to experience emotions and have self-reflection. Sometimes it's sadness, sometimes it's happiness, sometimes it's anger, sometimes it's resentment, sometimes it's grief, sometimes it's simply pure joy and love and feeling proud, no matter what, every single time it is healing.

Over time I realized how important it is to trust Peg as my therapist and life counselor. I also learned that the most beneficial sessions come from being raw and organic with myself. I really had to learn to trust myself, and love myself, and continue to choose to be honest with myself.

The ventral vagal state is where a person will experience self-reflection, joy, love, pride, and trust.

Healing from the Depths of My Heart and Soul

Jane, who weighed in on her sessions previously, wanted to make sure I concluded with this.

IFSsandtray was profound in my healing from the depths of my heart and soul. That's what's going through my head. Sandtray involved my heart and soul. I don't know how to describe it any other way. Something takes over. I don't even know, it's the Parts, it's personal. It's more personal to the inside of me than sandplay. I don't know when I was touching the sand and moving it around … it had to do with instinct. When I put the things in the sandtray. It's personal. It's the interior. It's something, it's something that's not represented. It's me, it's me and the feelings are in there, it's my insides it's my guts … Sandtray was very powerful for me. It took me to a different place.

Sandtray therapy integrated everything for me. I was in talk therapy for years. The changes I have made by doing therapy with you and working with sandtray were profound. They would have not been able to take place without the sand. The changes took place on a different level and again, on a soul level. My interior, psyche, whatever, it's inside and making it work. As opposed to other modes of therapy that have not moved it. It moved things. I am more empowered now. I am in a different place now.

In ending this chapter, I will go back to Cleopatra's written words that sum up what helping clients means to me, to many of my clients, and again I couldn't have said it better. She wrote:

Each day we have to "trust the process" and know that our journey is not about the finish line, rather about our current day, showing up for ourselves, and going full circle from trauma to healing.

Conclusion

18

Beginner's Mind in Trusting the Process

This book was born out of passion, love of current information for the treatment of complex psychological trauma, and curiosity. Or so I thought. More likely, I can attribute it to one of my own Parts and Pro-Symptom Beliefs of not feeling good enough. As one of the first, maybe the *only* American Association of Sex Educators Counselors and Therapists (AASECT) sex therapy supervisors in the year 2023—who has *also* been trained as a Registered Sandplay Practitioner (RSP) as well as certified in Internal Family Systems (IFS) therapist, and other modalities—I "should" know better. Alas, my multi-discipline training does not make me immune to everyday feelings.

Fortunately, all Parts have positive intentions and this one was no different. This Part, formed when I was a child in a loud, bustling family, was indeed young. It believed it could help me by filling a never-ending cycle of learning to be good enough. It took years for that Part to heal and spontaneously unburden after my own sandplay process was completed. The Part did take a new role, helping me feel "good enough" and changing my life completely. The Part now had a new role! One that inspired me to get a doctorate, and became instrumental in how this book was conceived and created.

Very early in this book I asked professional readers to have a beginner's mind—to trust in the latest up-to-date concepts in the field of psychotherapy in addressing psychological trauma, mental health, and sexual issues. Some of the concepts I introduce may seem foreign, even strange. For instance, the concept that all people have Parts, Parts that hold somatic sensations in *their bodies*, and are

DOI: 10.4324/9781003388302-22

protecting the client may sound preposterous. And yet, that concept has changed the lives of many clinicians and individuals, including many of my own clients and, indeed, colleagues. These peers have shared with me how their client's healing with IFS combined with other modalities is successful. Also, those clinicians trained in the Polyvagal Theory and IFS recognize how any person with a dysregulated autonomic nervous system can't be calm or, what IFS calls Self and in the Polyvagal Theory, is known as the ventral vagal state. Paying attention to the dysregulated autonomic nervous system helps both clinician and client.

Many of these well-trained peers accepted the importance of keeping an open mind. All of them were searching for techniques and cutting-edge modalities to incorporate into their therapeutic toolkits. During the advanced training, many of these well-educated individuals shared with me how they felt these new techniques seemed foreign and weird, and wondered whether they could master these very techniques. It may take months and years to gain a comprehensive knowledge of these new concepts, but with a dedicated mindset, many colleagues took the opportunity to learn something new and saw the results with their own clients.

An open mind will help you, the reader, better understand the new tools discussed within the pages of this book. Many of you may not have known the differences between sandtray or sandplay or the Pro-Symptom Belief Cards (PSBC). In addition, an introduction of sand and metaphor—as well as the PSBC—to heal trauma, mental, and sexual health disorders does feel unusual, far from the long conversations of talk therapy. But we are getting down to the unconscious. When a therapist witnesses the psyche and unconscious mind healing both physical and mental health issues from the inside out, we can attest to the real results. Just look at the cases of Betty, Billy, and Jane. Whereas years of talk therapy could only take them so far, they ultimately healed with IFSsandtray, Sandplay, and the PSBC. And in the case of Betty, who didn't have a sexual issue, working in both the sand and with the cards proved instrumental in navigating her early childhood trauma.

Sir Isaac Newton, among several early philosophers, used the phrase, "standing on the shoulders of giants." Like every professional, I have been influenced by the psychological masters of the past century as well as the influential mental health leaders of the last few decades. Sigmund Freud is often referred to as the "father of modern psychology;" and it's undeniable. All mental health professionals, no matter what modality they are trained, in stem from his original thinking and work.

And yet, it was Carl Gustav Jung, who—in breaking away from Freud's doctrine—added a new dimension to psychotherapy. The initial split, both philosophically and physically, caused significant psychological pain. But through his pain, and his vulnerability, Jung began his search for wholeness in an attempt to understand himself. He discovered having two personalities, number one, and number two, number one personality was dealing with the external world whereas the number two personality inhabited his inner world. These two personalities conflicted with each other; number one caused his depression while in number two he found great comfort. Without knowing it, he may have been the first person to discover Parts. Jung allowed himself to think creatively, resulting in his founding a new therapeutic modality. Jung's student, Dora Kalff the founder of sandplay modal, and an original thinker in her own right followed creative masters that went before her. It's an endless list.

Creativity in psychotherapy continues to be found in all the great master innovators of the past few decades. I have recognized tremendous creativity and insight in the creators of the newer modalities, like Internal Family Systems by Dr. Richard Schwartz, Sensorimotor Psychotherapy by Dr. Pat Ogden, and rethinking sex addiction by Doug Braun-Harvey and Michael Vigorito. The list continues with the sandplay researcher Dr. Lorraine Freedle who integrated the work of other master thinkers, Dr. Antonio Demasio and Dr. Bruce Perry's Neurosequential Model and Sandplay Therapy her chart is displayed in chapter eight. In addition, the pioneering and groundbreaking point of view of Dr. Gabor Mate and Dr. Stephen Porges' Polyvagal Theory. These are the broad shoulders I stand on and I have been able to tell a few of these innovative creative individuals how personally grateful I am for their mentorship which informed my own creativity and visions. My biggest vision when I wrote this textbook was to invite professionals to check their therapeutic tool kits, and their own Parts, and maybe even learn something new.

To this day, I stand in awe of the creative possibilities before me. I have not only stood on the shoulders of giants but looked ahead, into a future filled with possibilities. I look forward to new innovations in the field of healing, and vow to remain open, keeping a beginner's mind. It does take vulnerability for any clinician to go into in-depth training or treatment to find their own wounds. How can they expect their clients to do in-depth therapy when they haven't been open to themselves?

When clinician and client delve into the depths of the unconscious, innovation, creativity, and change occur naturally. It is imperative the clinician embrace, attune, quietly hold space, sit without hearing words, and witness the unconscious at work—allowing healing from the inside out. It takes a village, this is the power of the unconscious, Parts, and working with figurines and sand.

It seemed fitting to me to end this book with a quote from one of the greatest thinkers of our time, Albert Einstein.

"I have no special talent. I am only passionately curious."

Index

For Product Safety Concerns and Information please contact our EU
representative GPSR@taylorandfrancis.com
Taylor & Francis Verlag GmbH, Kaufingerstraße 24, 80331 München, Germany

9 7 8 1 0 3 2 4 8 2 9 1 0